THIS BOOK IS DEDICATED
TO ALL WOMEN
AND TO THE PURSUIT OF THEIR
LIMITLESS POTENTIAL.

DAYLE HADDON

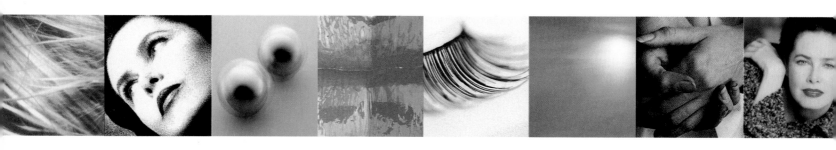

AGELESS BEAUTY

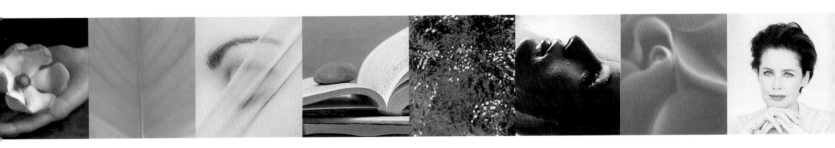

A WOMAN'S GUIDE TO LIFELONG BEAUTY AND WELL-BEING

HYPERION
NEW YORK

COPYRIGHT ©1998 DAYLE HADDON CONCEPTS

ALL RIGHTS RESERVED. NO PART OF THIS BOOK MAY BE USED
OR REPRODUCED IN ANY MANNER WHATSOEVER WITHOUT THE
WRITTEN PERMISSION OF THE PUBLISHER.
PRINTED IN THE UNITED STATES OF AMERICA.
FOR INFORMATION ADDRESS: HYPERION,
114 FIFTH AVENUE, NEW YORK, NEW YORK 10011.

LIBRARY OF CONGRESS CATALOGING-IN-PUBLICATION DATA
ISBN 0-7868-0445-1
FIRST EDITION
10 9 8 7 6 5 4 3 2 1

EDITOR: JENNIFER BARTH
CREATIVE DIRECTOR: GIOVANNI RUSSO/NO.11
ART DIRECTOR: MICHAEL ENGLISH
PHOTO EDITOR: BETH TAUBNER

ACKNOWLEDGEMENTS

I WOULD LIKE TO THANK CONNIE CLAUSEN FOR HER TREMENDOUS SPIRIT AND HER ENTHUSIASM FOR THIS BOOK FROM THE BEGINNING. STEDMAN MAYS WHO CARRIED ON WITH HIS UNIQUE ELEGANCE AND HUMOR THROUGH THE DAY-TO-DAY PROCESS, JENNIFER BARTH FOR HER BELIEF IN THE BOOK AND FOR HER SUPPORT IN CARRYING IT OUT. GIOVANNI RUSSO FOR SHARING MY VISION AND FOR HIS ENTHUSIASM AND WONDERFUL TALENT THAT BROUGHT THAT VISION TO LIFE, MICHAEL ENGLISH FOR HIS TIRELESS EXCITEMENT CREATING THE BOOK, JO FAIRLEY FOR HER ENDLESS CONTRIBUTIONS AND OUR MANY TRANSATLANTIC ADVENTURES, RUSTY PIERCE FOR HER GENEROUS INSIGHTS, ERICA PENN FOR HER PERSISTENCE IN REINFORCING THE RIGHT BALANCE, AND EMILY HARRISON, MY ALWAYS POSITIVE, RIGHT-HAND GIRL FRIDAY (AMONG EVERYTHING ELSE!) WHO KEPT ALL THE ELEMENTS AND PEOPLE TOGETHER AND HAPPY. I THANK YOU A MILLION TIMES.

TO MY GUARDIAN ANGEL RAY, WHO HELPED TURN MY LIFE AROUND 180 DEGREES AND TO WHOM I OWE SO MUCH, AND MY SECOND ANGEL, DAVE ROY, WHOSE KINDNESS OF SPIRIT IS MATCHED BY HIS INFINITE WISDOM.

I EXTEND MY GRATITUDE FOR THE UNENDING BELIEF, ENTHUSIASM AND SUPPORT THROUGHOUT THE DEVELOPMENT OF THIS BOOK FROM MICHAEL SPIESSBACH AND SAM WAKSAL, NO MATTER WHERE THEY WERE IN THE WORLD.

I THANK THE WARMTH AND SUPPORT OF MY L'ORÉAL TEAM BECAUSE "THEY ARE WORTH IT":
LINDSEY OWEN-JONES, PATRICK RABAIN, GUY PERLONGUE, JOE CAMPINELL, CAROL HAMILTON,
FABRICE BOÉ-DREYFUS, AND ALL THE TALANTED GANG THERE.

TO JACK SCHNEIDER FOR HIS AMAZING SUPPORT THROUGHOUT.
TO DAN STERN FOR HIS IMMEDIATE BELIEF AND CREATIVITY.
TO DAN LUFKIN FOR THE SUPPORT SO EARLY ON.
TO BERT FIELDS FOR HIS GENEROUS EXPERTISE AND FRIENDSHIP.
TO MY DEAR BRYAN BANTRY, WHO FROM DAY ONE CHAMPIONED FOR HIS WOMEN AND JENNIFER HARRIS WHO CARRIED THE IDEA OUT WONDERFULLY, DAY IN AND DAY OUT.
TO LEONARD LAUDER AND BOB LUZZI FOR THEIR HELP AND GENEROSITY.
FOR THE ONGOING SUPPORT, KNOWLEDGE, AND EXPERTISE OF LARRY DARBY.
THE EXTRA EFFORTS ON THE PART OF ALAN GOLDBERG.
FOR THE EXQUISITE MAKEUP MAGIC OF SANDY LINTER THAT HAS TRANSFORMED ME OVER THE YEARS.
TO PATRICK DEMARCHELIER FOR HIS ENDLESS HELP AND THE GENEROUS EFFORTS OF MICHEL COMTE AND TROY WORD.

TO MICHELE BERNHARDT FOR HER AMAZING INSIGHTS, HER SWEETNESS OF SPIRIT, AND HER EXTRAORDINARY FRIENDSHIP OVER THE YEARS, AND REGINA KULIK FOR THE ENCOURAGEMENT, THE LOVE, THE ADVICE, AND THE ENDLESS LAUGHTER.

I AM GRATEFUL FOR THE UNCONDITIONAL LOVE OF MY FAMILY; THE WELL FROM WHICH I CONSTANTLY DRAW, AND FOR MY DAUGHTER, RYAN, WHO DAILY REFLECTS THE GIFTS AND CHALLENGES OF INNER AND OUTER BEAUTY.

I THANK ALL MY FRIENDS FOR THEIR PATIENCE AND UNDERSTANDING OF MY LONG ABSENCE DURING THE CREATION OF THIS BOOK! AT EACH MOMENT OF THIS ADVENTURE, THEY BUOYED ME UP WITH AN ENCOURAGING WORD, ENTHUSIASTIC RESPONSE, AMD A SYMPATHETIC EAR THAT MADE ME GO FARTHER THAN I THOUGHT ON THEIR SUPPORT AND LOVE.

AND, TO ALL OF THE PHOTOGRAPHERS, STYLISTS, MAKEUP ARTISTS, AND HAIRDRESSERS I HAVE WORKED WITH OVER THE LAST THIRTY PLUS YEARS, I THANK YOU FOR THE FRIENDSHIPS, THE FUN, AND FOR EVERYTHING I HAVE LEARNED IN THIS BUSINESS FROM EACH ONE OF YOU.

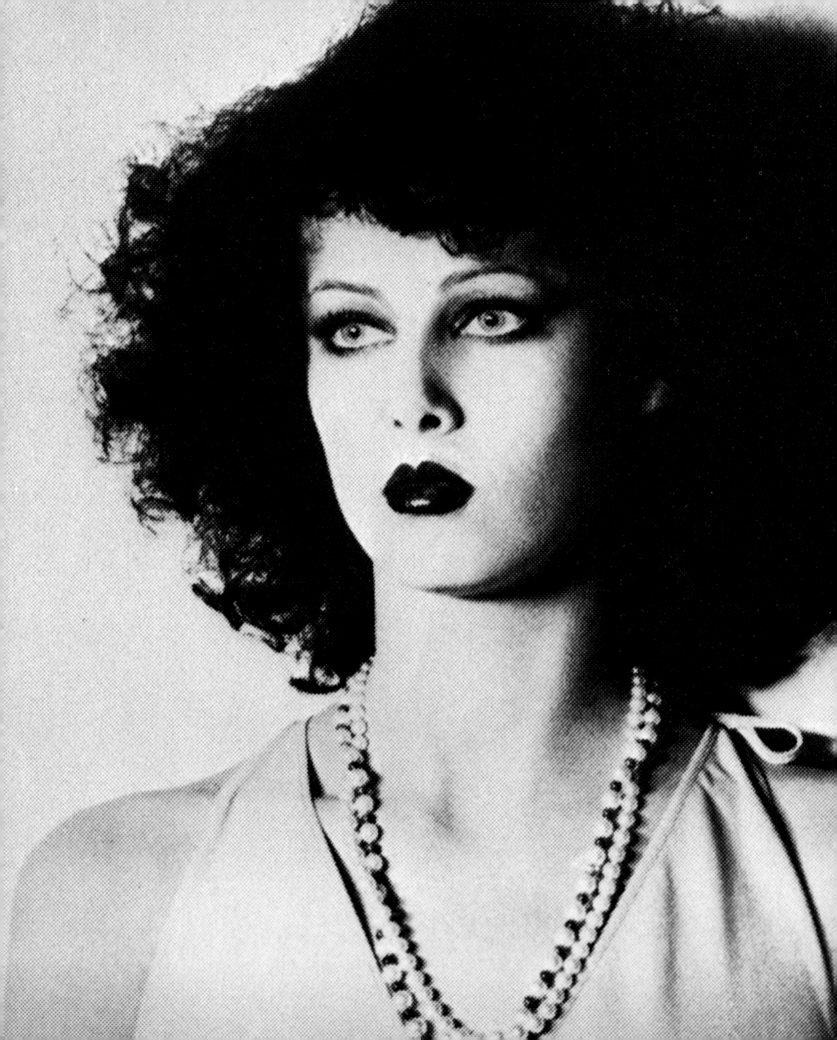

photograph by Guy Bourdin, *French Vogue*, 1974

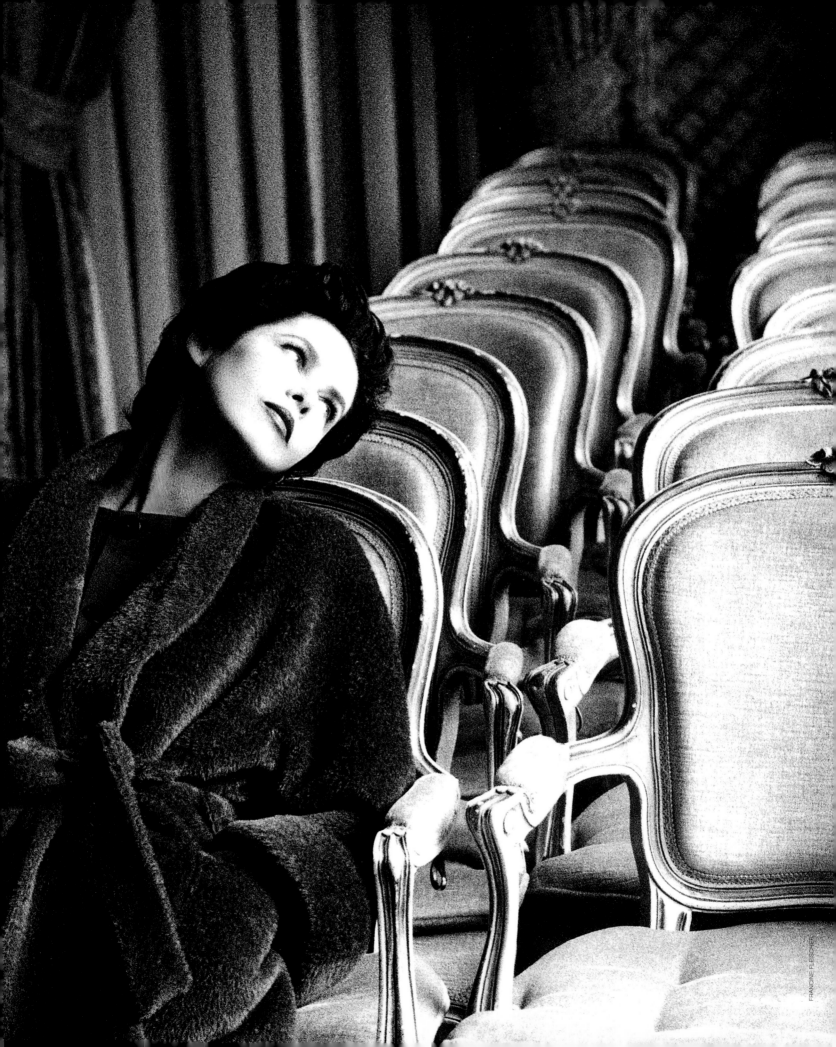

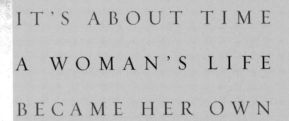

IT'S ABOUT TIME
A WOMAN'S LIFE
BECAME HER OWN

Ten years ago, my husband died suddenly, leaving me to raise my fifteen-year-old daughter alone. In a heartbeat, I lost almost everything: my partner, my home, my security.

I had to start over. I desperately wanted my daughter, Ryan, to be able to have the possibilities a college education would offer her. Financially depleted, I had to find work right away. But what were my qualifications? The only things I knew were modeling and acting, but when I tried to find work in either of these professions again, the doors started slamming in my face. "You're past it." "You're too old." "Thanks, but no thanks." I was basically being told that my life was over. But I wasn't ready to walk into the sunset anytime soon.

I could no longer afford to live in my house, so I rented it out and moved into a small maid's room off a friend's kitchen that was kindly offered. I had my daughter to support, so I still had to find a job. Having no luck in my own business, I didn't know what I could do. I thought about waitressing, but after getting up my courage to put in an application at a nearby restaurant, to my shock, I was turned down. I tried a few other avenues but couldn't seem to get anything off the ground; somehow, a grieving woman was like a bad luck charm. Except for a few close friends, nobody had the time for my difficulties. It felt as if I was standing still and everyone else was rushing past me. I realized I was not going to be "saved." I had to save myself.

Eventually, through a friend of a friend of a friend, I managed to secure a position in one of the small advertising agencies dotted around L.A., making coffee, washing dishes, answering phones. But I was thrilled to get it: It was a job.

I was still trying for parts in movies (and not getting them). With my scripts precariously balanced on my knees beneath my desk, I waited for a lull in the phone calls to study my roles. I squeezed time during my lunch break to go on auditions, rushing back before my employers noticed I was gone.

I was faxing and FedExing, washing up and making a mean cup of coffee. I was also learning a lot of organizational skills that would serve me well later on. But all this was not going to put my daughter through college—or get me out of the maid's room. Something had to change.

One day, as I was routinely filing the week's documents, I stopped dead in my tracks. Viewing the agency's budget, I discovered the coyote in the Dodge commercial the agency was filming earned more money than I did. It was time to move on. Time to move up to the next level of my life.

But fate had a few more surprises in store for me. My tenants had trashed my house. The real estate agent stated that in all her years of experience, she'd never seen a rental left in worse shape—dog-chewed furniture, smashed treasures, torn curtains. Sorting through the half-eaten objects, I spied the treasured wooden duck I had discovered long ago at a flea market. The entire head had been chewed off in some canine frenzy. As I surveyed the wreckage of my home, I realized I'd hit rock bottom.

I had never been a practical or efficient person, and I certainly did not know anything about duck-head replacing. But it was either give up or fight back. I decided to start right there. I flipped through the Yellow Pages—nothing under "Damaged Duck Heads" or "Canine Catastrophes." After an extensive search I discovered a kindly furniture restorer who restored my faith in mankind when he smiled and responded, "Yes, I think we can fix this." I had solved the problem. This insignificant event was a turning point for me. If I could mend the duck, it meant I could probably mend my life. I attacked the rest of the destruction piece by piece, learning, growing, and winning along the way.

Energized and optimistic, I realized I had so much to offer—even if the world didn't happen to agree. I decided to hit the library and start researching the statistics about women of my generation—the baby boomers—and my discoveries amazed me. The fastest growing chunk of the population was women between forty-five and fifty-five. In the next couple of years forty million women were going to reach their forties. Wow. That's me. That's us. But who was listening? Or speaking up for us? I certainly wasn't about to accept that only the first part of my life had any real value.

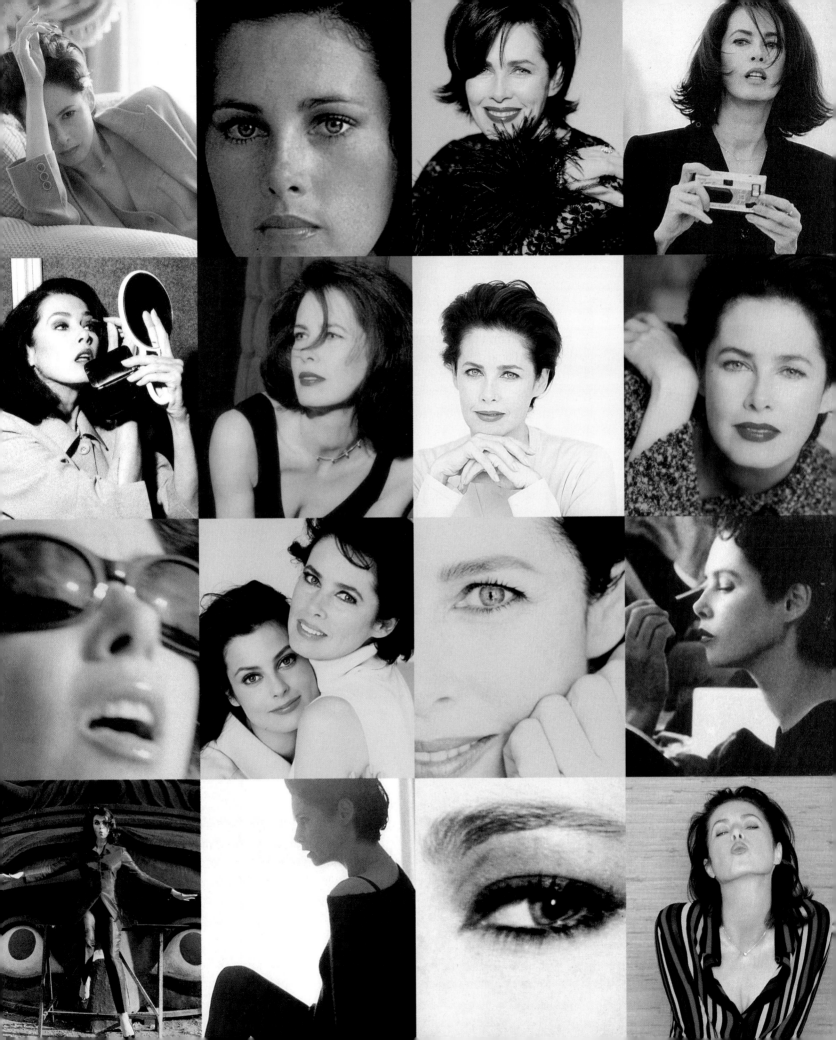

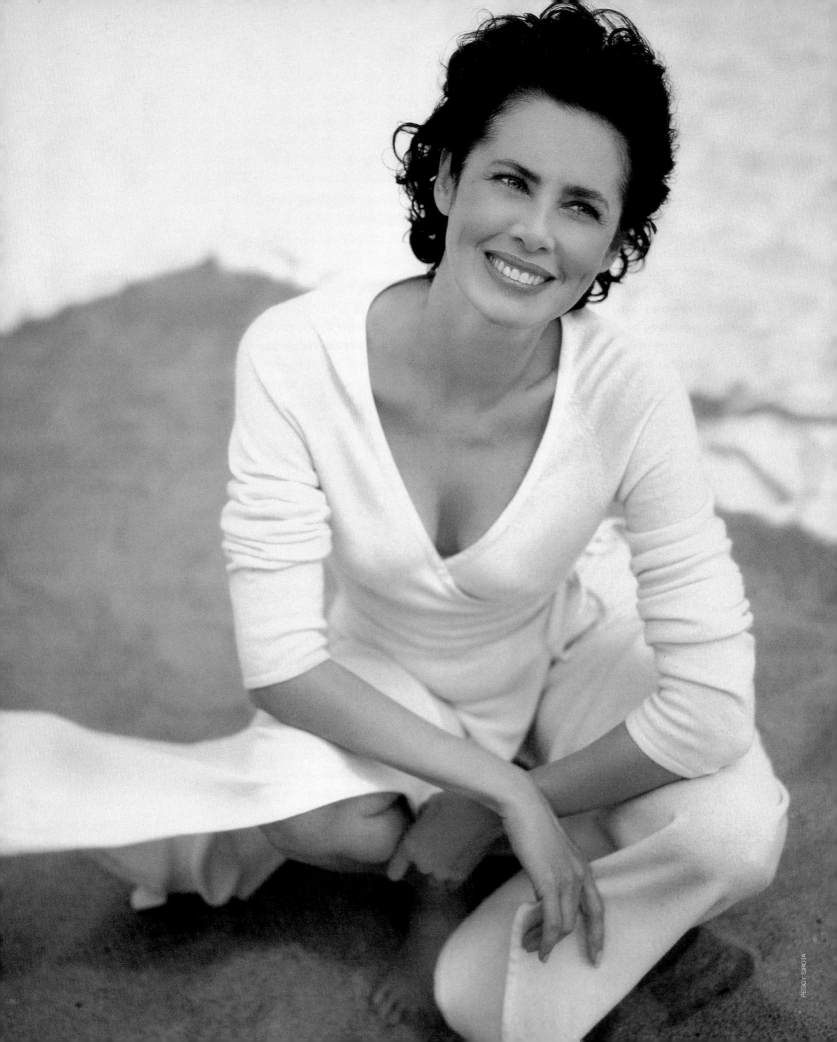

I scoured through my Rolodex and started knocking on doors of the major cosmetics companies to tell them they were really missing something. By only focusing on fresh-faced teenagers and twentysomethings, they were neglecting a vast number of women on this planet like me, like my friends. Again I had doors slammed in my face—but I didn't give up.

For me, "no" doesn't mean no—it means maybe. I had a real conviction that I was right, which gives great strength in any situation. I asked them: What are you going to do for the millions of women over forty who feel great, look better than ever, but want even more? Why aren't these women being portrayed in the media? Why aren't you talking to the enormous number of women out there? And the more I spoke to women of my generation, the more I realized how upset they were about not being represented in magazines or the media. They felt invisible. They felt devalued and they didn't like it one bit. Neither did I.

I persevered in the face of rejection. Bit by bit, the doors slowly began to open; the cosmetics executives began to sit up and listen. It was a new idea, to show the continuity between the beauty of youth *and* the evolution of true beauty that only years of experience can bring; the idea that beauty never ends and is certainly not the exclusive property of the young.

With my friend and agent, Bryan Bantry, I helped start up a revolutionary model agency that began with two older models—one of them me—and now has thirty-five of us on the books. Ten years ago, our careers would have been finished. Not anymore.

Then, the breakthrough: first Clairol, who shattered the age barrier by featuring top models of the '70s and '80s on a major hair color line, selected me as a spokesperson. Next, I was chosen to be the face of a new anti-aging line for Estée Lauder. Then, the exact day that the Lauder contract expired, L'Oréal jumped in and signed me up. Working with L'Oréal, I've been able to do what I really love: travel the world and meet women with real-life concerns and real-life dreams. And by choosing me as their "face" for the skin-care line Plénitude, L'Oréal is celebrating the dawn of a new age for woman in which nobody minds how old you are.

I have always been a woman's woman; in this so-called man's world, I feel a bond with women: empathy, sympathy, camaraderie, and admiration. I believe it is time to establish a new blueprint for aging, one that acknowledges and applauds our enduring value and celebrates what we have gained, not what we have lost. Ask any woman over forty: Would you want the insecurities of being twenty-three again? No way! So a few lines and wrinkles are a small tradeoff for the knowledge, the wisdom, the confidence that only comes with age. I love the fact that my face is the face I have earned.

Throughout the thirty years of my career, I've had the good fortune to have worked with some of the greatest photographers (from Horst to Beaton, Avedon to Lartigue), as well as the very best makeup artists, hairdressers, and stylists. Although I don't look like the stereotypical model and have never considered myself sidewalk-stopping beautiful, women have constantly asked me for beauty secrets. I believe that beauty comes from within. It is a belief that I have always developed and nurtured. My success has been more about who I am than what I look like. I love when other women teach me, and I'm happy to share what I know: from fat-busting exercises to energy boosters, from makeup tricks to finding a perfect age-appropriate style. I especially love those little time-saving tips that can shave minutes off your day and hours off your week, freeing up time to do what makes you smile. In fact, when I ask almost any '90s woman what she'd like more of, time is always at the top of her wish list.

I felt compelled to write this book because I wanted to share with women everywhere ways we can find that elusive quality: balance. It's a fact of life: We all know that how we look has a direct influence on how we feel. But then there's the bigger stuff: how to get through those times when you think you'll never feel great about anything again; how to have more joy, more spirituality, an inner life—as well as handle the constant stream of stuff. This is the challenge of day-to-day life, for all of us, as we hurtle toward the new millennium.

My life hasn't always been handed to me. It took me ten years just to get my career off the ground: I was told I was too small, didn't look right, and wasn't wanted. Eventually, I was "discovered." I found success and took off—and I had some great years. Then the shock. After losing my husband, it took what seemed like forever to get back on my feet again. The climb back up was not a straight path, but I owe so much of who I am today to that journey. We have the lean times and then it's great again. This is the roller coaster called life.

There are some dramatic curveballs that life can throw a woman. Midlife often involves saying good-bye to people who have meant a great deal to us. It means coming to terms with—and letting go of—things that once were important. Sometimes we must also "let go" of the person we were in order to discover who we can become. I often say to women: "This is your movie—you decide what's going to happen next." While we do not control most of the larger events in our lives, we can control our attitude toward them. And I honestly believe: The greater the pain, the greater the treasure. As a result of all the obstacles I've encountered, I know I have more compassion, more humor, more gratitude, more enthusiasm, more understanding, a greater sense of my own value, and a deep appreciation for the infinite, glorious value of life.

There has never been a better time in history for a woman over forty—if we get it right. Armed with information about advances in science, medicine, cosmetics, psychology, technology, we are on the threshold of a life that has never been available before, a life in which we don't have to kiss good-bye to our sexuality, sensuality, health, fitness, well-being, or good looks simply because of a meaningless date on our driver's license. We can be strong and sexy. Powerful and pretty. Focused and feminine. This is an adventure. So won't you join me in the celebration?

"ONE IS NOT BORN A WOMAN,

ONE BECOMES ONE"

SIMONE DE BEAUVOIR

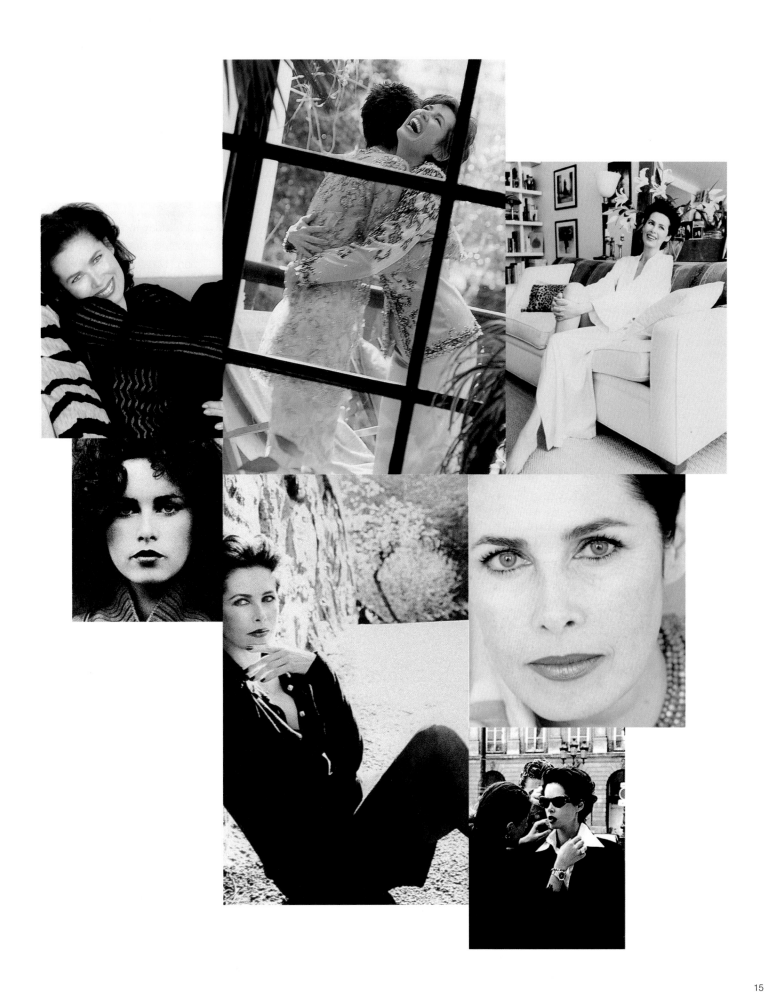

15

THE
AGEQUAKE

BECAUSE THE AGE WE ARE NOW IS THE BEST AGE EVER

The first wave of seventy-six million baby boomers has finally hit fifty. Over the next decade, our "class" of fiftysome-things will swell by 50 percent, making us the fastest-growing segment of the population. Just a few years ago, hitting forty meant you had reached your prime; it was all downhill from here. Not anymore. Now we are just awakening to the extraordinary possibilities of life opening up to us as this agequake shakes, rattles, and rocks our world.

At the turn of the century, a woman's life expectancy was somewhere in her forties. Now a woman of forty can often expect more than forty years ahead of her, and she's asking: How can I make the very most of this time? Medical and scientific advances have extended our lifespan and quality of living. At fifty, if she stays free from cancer and heart disease, a woman can reasonably expect to reach her ninety-second birthday.

It is time to redefine what it is to grow old. Forty isn't what it used to be, nor is fifty. What was old for our mothers is no longer old for us. When our baby boomer generation hits seventy, you can bet that we will redefine expectations about what seventy should look like, too. According to Ross Goldstein, a psychologist with the Generation Insights consulting firm, "It's going to be hip to be old."

Everywhere we look, we see examples of women demonstrating how great forty, fifty, and up can be. Over-forties are our cultural icons—not has-beens or gonna-bes. We have inspiring role models in politics, entertainment, the media, and business: Barbara Walters, Oprah Winfrey, Diane Sawyer, Maya Angelou, Bette Midler, Hillary Rodham Clinton, Tina Brown, Sherry Lansing, Goldie Hawn, Anjelica Huston, Martha Stewart, Cherie Blair, Sharon Stone, Donna Karan, Sophia Loren, Connie Chung, Susan Sarandon, Joanne Woodward, Barbra Streisand, Jill Barad, Gail Sheehy, Cher, Aretha Franklin, Meryl Streep, Gloria Steinem, Katie Couric, Toni Morrison, Marion Wright Edelman, Sandra Day O'Conner . . . to name a few!
A recent advertising campaign for Nike depicted a woman of fifty as representing "the age of elegance." In marketing terms, this is a 180 degree turn. Traditionally, the media and manufacturers targeted twentysomethings and thirtysomethings with messages about looking and feeling great. Older women were left to fend for themselves, assuming they would passively leave beauty and well-being behind with their youth. We simply will not accept that anymore. Today, we are hungry for information and products that will turbo-charge the quality of our lives, keeping us fabulous, fit, flexible, and fun-loving—both mentally and physically—forever. At the same time, after years of caring for a family or devoting ourselves to advancing a career, we are finally searching for much, much more: quality of life, simple joys, meaning, a sense of value, our own spirituality (not to mention our spectacles), and a renewed sense of self.

The new definition of beauty that goes hand-in-hand with this agequake embraces a harmony of inner and outer beauty—a merging of who you are with what you look like, an attitude that radiates health, wisdom, experience, energy, and joy. This is true beauty. Being a woman at midlife means you are at the center where can look back and draw from the past yet have a future to create ahead of you. Today this is about looking and feeling the best we can, irrespective of our age—no longer trying to live up to unrealistic ideals but celebrating who we are now. At the same time, we have never had more help. The cosmetics companies and fashion designers have awakened to the enormous financial clout that baby boomers wield. Anti-aging products, which are the fastest growing skincare category, deliver greater benefits than ever. In the wake of Donna Karan, the first in the fashion industry to acknowledge that we have womanly hips, tummies, and thighs, many designers are now creating for real bodies and real women, not runway nymphs. And because baby boomers have always been interested in being beautiful as well as smart, stylish as well as successful, sexy as well as savvy, we're not about to throw out our lash-building mascaras or our Wonderbras!

The sophisticated woman wants it all: to look good, feel great and have the tools and the time to achieve her true potential. None of us feels we have enough time. We want shortcuts—small lifestyle changes that will pay big dividends. We are creating a personal blueprint for the next thirty, forty, or fifty years of looking, feeling and being fabulous. It's not about selfishness: it's about selfness—achieving true well-being so that we have the most to offer ourselves and everyone around us.

So it is time to celebrate what we have gained—not what we have lost—over the years. This is the dawning of a wonderful new life. It isn't over. It's just beginning!

PART ONE

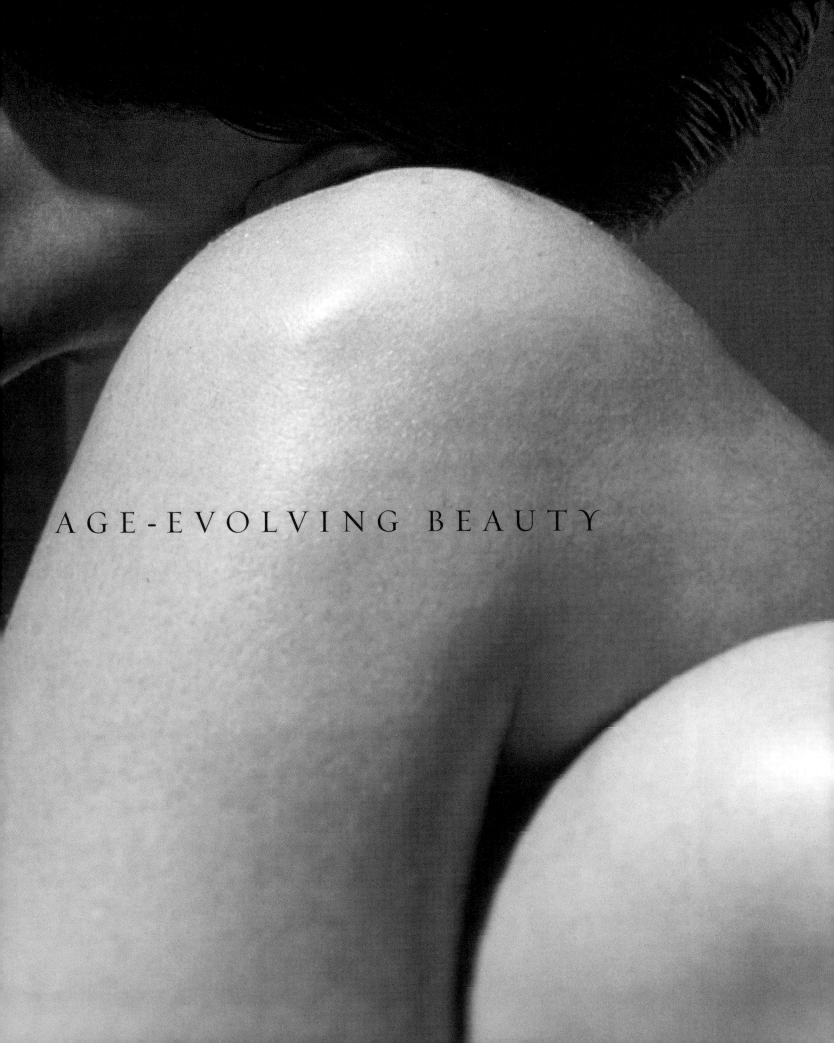

AGE-EVOLVING BEAUTY

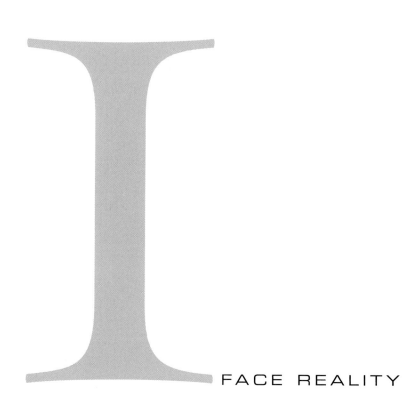

I

FACE REALITY

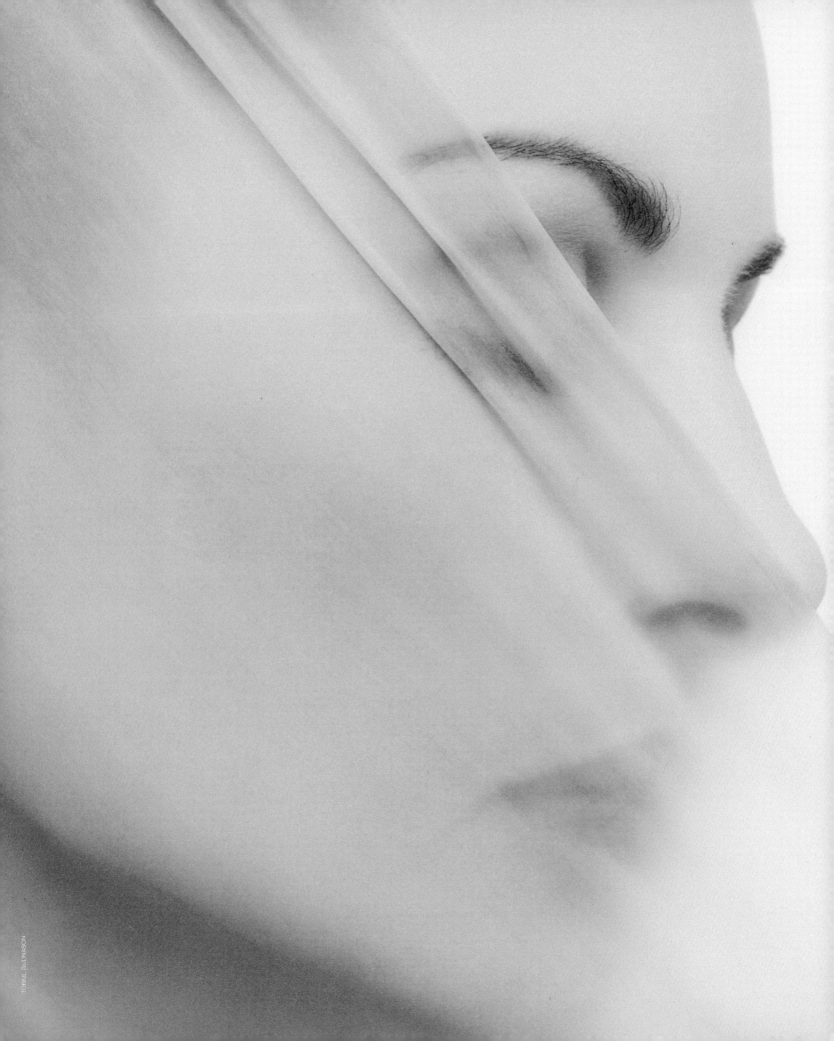

SKIN
THE BOTTOM LINE ON LINES

As we age, the changes in our skin worry many women. Suddenly, we don't have the skin we used to have; seeing our changed reflection staring back at us can make us feel old. We may be the same person inside as we were in our twenties—but what's staring back at us sends a very different message. As we age, it is natural and okay to develop lines and wrinkles and to realize that our skin doesn't recover as quickly as it once did. Over the years, sun, pollution, and bad eating habits have all done some damage, leaving our skin with special needs. The great news is that even if you've *never* properly cared for your skin before, now is the best time to start, taking advantage of the enormous advances recently made in skin-care technology.

The skin does much more than simply cover what's inside: it's the largest organ of the body. It breathes, excretes, absorbs, and protects. In fact, caring for your skin can be one of your most powerful weapons in the fight against aging, because the skin so quickly reflects back the TLC you lavish upon it.

There is nothing sexier than great skin. When you wake up in the morning, it may be all you're wearing, and you want it to be in tip-top shape . . . at whatever age. When you roll over and whisper, "Hello darling!"—even if it's just to your reflection in the mirror!—you want to love what is seen.

Much of human interaction is tactile; when someone shakes your hand on an introduction, touches your arm in acknowledgment, or tenderly caresses your face, it casts a strong impression of who you are. Does this contact with others reflect that you are taking good care of yourself? Is the feel of your skin giving off signs of neglect? If you nourish and care for your skin, you can have sensual skin all the way up through your seventies and eighties.

In our twenties, we thought we got away with murder: falling into bed without removing our makeup, skimping on skin care, baking in the sun. But it all catches up with us, and now we're at an age when we must nourish the skin. Serious nourishment. Our skin needs to be revitalized and pampered on a daily basis, with a skin-care ritual performed religiously, come rain, snow, sleet . . . or late nights.

COMING CLEANER Skin needs to breathe and rejuvenate itself each night; it needs to be entirely cleansed of makeup, cellular debris, and the grime we pick up from daily life. The skin's rate of cell renewal is at its highest at night, and the absorption of active-care products increases between midnight and 4 a.m. So, be sure to capitalize on this anti-aging opportunity.

I completely cleanse my face at night. For me, it's like washing away the stress of the day. It's my time to reflect on what happened during the day. But you must be extremely gentle with your skin. When cleansing and nourishing, always use gentle, outward motions; otherwise you can literally stretch the skin.

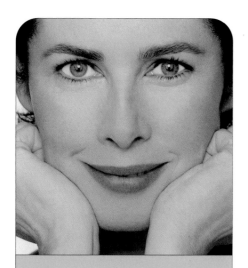

IT'S ABOUT TIME . . .

. . . to face reality. At this age, we've traded experience and wisdom for a few lines. I call that a bargain. Because today there is so much that we can do to brighten and tighten our faces, put back that youthful glow—and even reverse signs of aging. So let me share with you some of my wisdom—acquired behind the scenes in the world of skin care, beauty, and make-up over the course of more than thirty years. The secrets and tips that can help every woman look her very best.

Never rub, pull, or tug. Try to lightly pat, or use delicate gliding movements when caring for your skin.

When it comes to removing eye makeup, be especially careful. I always use a product specifically formulated to do the job. I think Lancôme's eye make-up remover is excellent. (Although, if I'm traveling, I might use good old Quickies pads, which you can get at the drugstore.) I apply the eye makeup remover to a Kleenex; I delicately cleanse the lid, then, holding the lashes between my "tis-sued" fingers, I softly roll the mascara back and forth until all of it comes off. Coax the makeup off your lashes, don't tug or you can pull them out. If you rub the eye area, you're disturbing the extremely fragile under-eye skin. The goal at all times is to minimize wear and tear.

Treat the face and neck as one, cleansing them both at the same time. (And don't forget the area under your hair at the back of the neck, which can accumulate grime during the day.) I'm from the splash-water-on-the-face school; cold water, in the morning, is particularly refreshing and really helps with early a.m puffiness.

SKIN TONIC As we age, alcohol in skin tonic becomes too drying for skin. Nevertheless, I love the fresh, tingling feeling of a tonic or a skin toner, which I feel removes every last trace of makeup. I look for one that's non-alcoholic. I like the smell and feel of L'Oréal Plénitude Toner. It is light and gentle, but cleanses deeply. I sweep a cotton pad, soaked in the tonic, over my face and all over my neck (front and back), and down toward my chest, too. Alternatively, I'll use rosewater, which you can find in most health food stores or pharmacies. It smells delicious and is very gentle, so it suits even the driest complexions. All this is foreplay, before we nourish.

DREAM CREAMS At this age, we have to moisturize, moisturize, moisturize. Skin has different needs now. It's thirstier, finer, more fragile. I cannot and should not use the same cream as my daughter. My creams are too heavy and rich for her skin—but mine drinks them up. At night I recommend using a cream that makes up for what the day has robbed from the skin. Revitalift Night is one of the terrific products in L'Oréal's Pléntitude line that I trust (and am proud to represent!). It contains a vitamin A derivative to fight wrinkles. For a light day cream, I recommend Lancôme Primordiale, which comes in a squirt bottle (squirt bottles are great because they prevent contamination caused by repeatedly dip-ping your fingers directly into a cream). Then I put a layer of sunblock over the top. (First, wait for the moisturizer to sink in, otherwise the sunblock spreads on too thinly.)

Treat your neck and décolletage as an extension of your face; the sun strikes this area without us even realizing it—especially in summer, with scoop necks and undone buttons. Katharine Hepburn always said she liked to wear turtlenecks to hide the appearance of her neck. In my experience, although the neck is vulnerable to aging, it doesn't have to sag. It helps to stand up straight and stretch regularly. Older women who practice yoga always seem to have the most fabulous necks and chins.

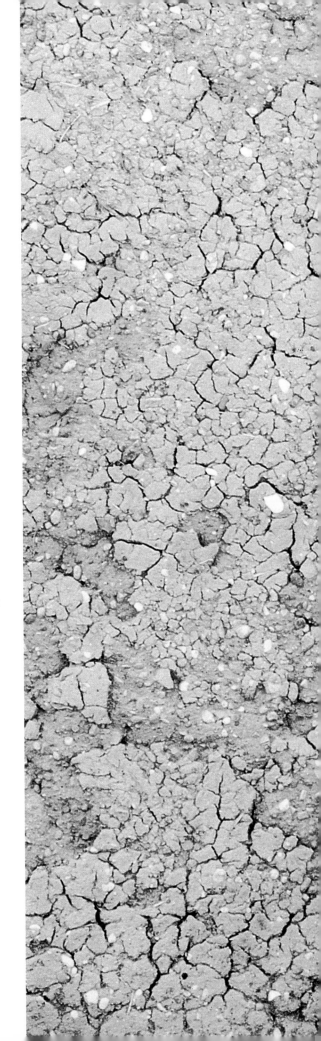

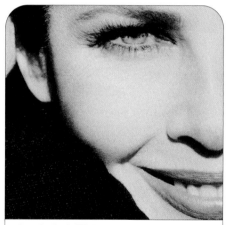
LAUGH LINES

Find your laugh lines:
To see where you should
apply your eye cream,
squinch up your eyes to see
how far the lines go. Be sure
to include *all* of this area
when you moisturize.

When applying moisturizer, never pull the skin. The muscle that runs from the jaw to the cheek is what tends to give out over time—so think up, up, up, patting, almost tapping upward along that muscle. Try to follow the line of the muscle where it's wrapped around the bone. Patting also stimulates circulation and can even ease stress. We all carry a lot of tension in the jaw and gentle patting can help diffuse it. (I remember going to a masseuse in Paris who worked with all the top French actresses—Catherine Deneuve, Anouk Aimée, Marie-Sophie Lelouch—and her signature was deep massage and patting of the jaw. If these great-looking women are anything to go by, I figured she must be on to something.)

THE RETIN-A QUESTION I'm not a fan of Retin-A, although I have seen tremendous differences in some women who have used it. Retin-A is a strong, vitamin A-based prescription-only treatment. Originally developed for acne sufferers, it was found to be effective as an anti-aging treatment, reducing the depth of wrinkles, lightening age spots, and "brightening" skin. But it has to be used for a long period of time—usually a year, minimum—and makes skin very sun-sensitive. I don't like the fact that using retin-A makes skin so vulnerable to the sun. I also don't like to be such a slave to a particular treatment, ball-and-chained to a cream. If you do decide to go for Retin-A, though, my advice is to take special care of your neck. I see women who use the cream and achieve very smooth faces; but their necks give them away. Remember, face and neck should be treated as one!

EYES RIGHT The skin under the eyes is finer and more fragile than the rest of the face. Because it has fewer oil glands, the skin around the eyes is more prone to wrinkling. I like to dab on my eye cream in a line around the socket above and below the eyes. You don't need to put the cream directly under the eye, because it does travel to where it's needed. (This way you can minimize sensitivity problems, too.) Be sure to include all of the area that extends from the eye outward to the hairline—the laugh-line area. Make sure this area is very well moisturized. We want you to be fearless about laughter!

Find your laugh lines: To see where you should apply your eye cream, squinch up your eyes to see how far the lines go. Be sure to include all of this area when you moisturize.

SUN PROTECTION SECRETS I choose to stroll down the shady side of the street; I put towels over my body if I'm near the sun; I pull my sleeves down over my hands if I happen to be walking in the sun. I would wear gloves and carry a parasol if I could get away with it! I make do with a collection of wide-brimmed hats in every size, shape, and color. I also have collapsible versions, made by Eric Javits, that fit in my bag and are smart, safe, and chic. I even swim in them (see Resources). And there's no way, José, that I'm going to leave the house without sunblock. I think the sun is life-giving; I love spring sun and winter sun, but I never go out without protection between April and

November, because the sun is truly the greatest cause of premature aging known to women. I would wear SPF 1,000,000 if it were available. Instead, I make do with SPF 30 (a favorite is Chritstian Dior's UV30 for face), applied about fifteen minutes after my moisturizer, so it has time to sink in. For women who want a physical sun block as opposed to a sunscreen, Nutrogena's Sensitive Skin SPF17 is a great choice because it doesn't cause skin irritation. I keep little tubes of sunblock in my handbag, in the car, on my desk—to remind me to use it. Remember: Even with an SPF, you will still develop some color through the sun-block, but more gradually, and without the burn and skin damage.

Try to get in the habit of rubbing whatever sunblock is left over the tops of your hands. The darker brown–pigmented spots that develop there, called "age spots," are a real age giveaway—and they're almost exclusively a result of sun exposure. If you protect your hands from additional exposure, these may gradually fade.

SKIN BRIGHTENING   It's a fact of life that as we age, skin cell turnover slows down, which is one reason why the older we get, the duller, dingi-er, and sometimes even grayer our skin looks. The best treatment for this is exfo-liation. I don't necessarily use a special exfoliant—but I do slough away dead surface skin cells on my face with a thin, nubby terry cloth towel. Don't rub—or you'll end up with broken blood vessels (whether you're nineteen or ninety). Simply buff the skin, ultralightly, in little circular skimming movements. You can apply a little more pressure in the creases on both sides of the nose and on the chin, where skin cells build up fastest and where blackheads can develop. Avoid buffing around the under-eye area, which is too fragile.

Every now and then I will use an exfoliant for my skin, like L'Oréal's Excell–A3. I like to use this sort of product about once a month, when my skin looks tired. I find that it gives me a wonderful skin-brightening effect with just one treatment. Alternatively, I'll use a clay-based mask, applying it to my neck, face, and chest, and then I'll jump in the shower to rinse it off, intensively moistur-izing afterward. Because the surface skin cells have been removed, moisturizers can penetrate more deeply. The entire effect is terrific!

NO MORE FROWN LINES   Over time, our faces tend to devel-op bad habits: frowning and squinting. But it isn't impossible to change these habits of a lifetime, if you become conscious of them. The other day, I was meeting with a beautiful top executive, noticing that as she talked, her forehead was pleated with worry lines. It was distracting and prematurely aging. Another friend is guilty of not wearing the glasses she needs, so her constant squint, as she strains to see, has now become almost a permanent expression. The first thing to do is to become aware of your bad expression habits. Ask a friend to point them out to you. There are many ways to beat the problem. You might try good old "Frownies," which are stick-on patches that make it difficult to frown (see resources). Another trick is a regular, soothing facial massage, which melts the tension from the face. You can even do it yourself for a few seconds, several times a day: Simply make delicate stroking movements along the brow, working from the center out.

TIP

If you drive a lot during the summer months, make sure that you use sunblock on your hands and face (espe-cially the left side), wear a hat and, if possible, have tinted-glass car windows.

TIP

A new approach to reduce wrinkles is a powerful anti-oxidant, ascorbic acid (it works much like Retin-A).

"WE
OURSELVES
POSSESS BEAUTY
WHEN WE
ARE TRUE TO
OUR OWN
BEING"

PLOTINUS

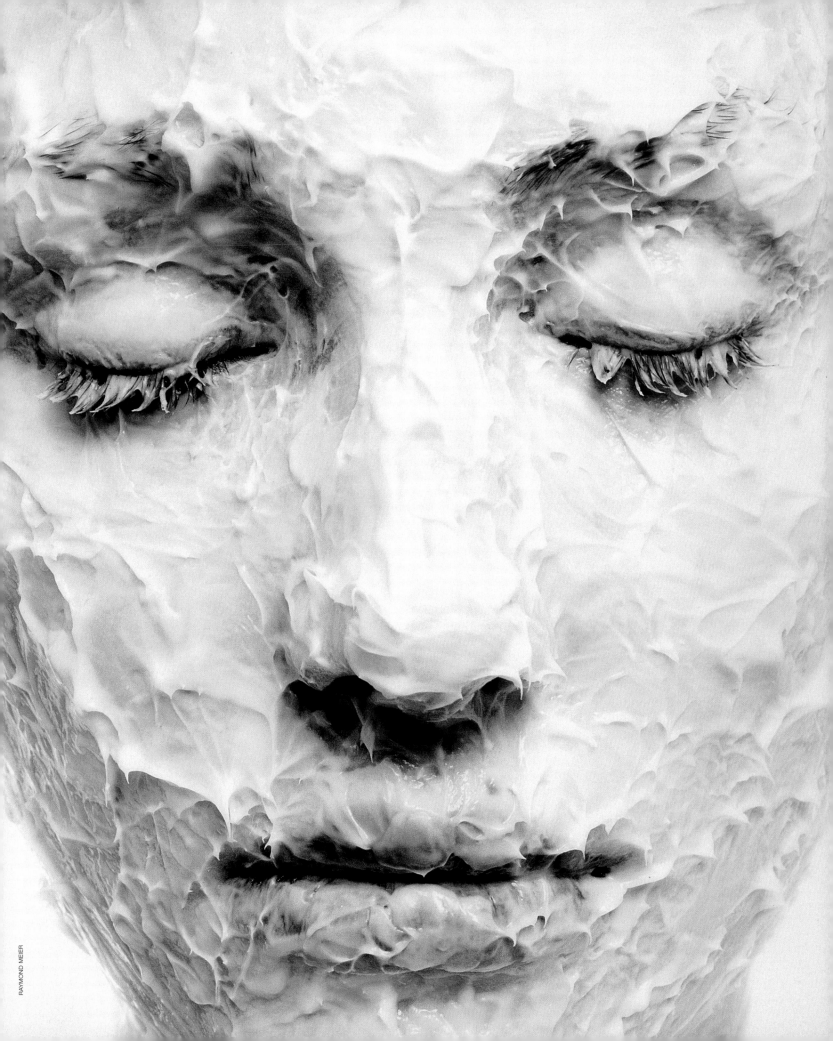

Alternatively—and this might sound wacky, but it works—rub your hands together to create warmth. Hold your hands together, as if you were cupping them around a ball; you'll almost feel a buzz of electricity as you bring the fingers together. Raise your hands to cover your face and hover over the surface of your skin as you smooth the forehead, traveling up and over the hairline, across the cheekbones, and outward along the jawline. Experience the heat and energy from your fingers, before you physically touch your face. This can be incredibly relaxing. Another trick is to stroke the top of your head with a light touch.

A light, tapping facial massage can also relax the face and diminish frown lines. (I personally believe that the skin is like a sheet; if left, over time, without further crumpling, then creases will release and eventually disappear.) With your ring finger, tap from the chin upward, across the sinus area, and around the eye socket, in a circular movement.

A modern-day, increasingly popular alternative is Botox, which when injected paralyzes the muscles of the face for a period of months, therefore "re-training" the expression (see Nips and Tucks, p. 47).

MOISTURE POWER   We spend so much time and money applying moisturizing creams to our skin, but we often forget to moisturize the environment we live in. During wintertime, or in heated or air-conditioned rooms, the humidity level plunges to that of the Sahara, literally sucking moisture from our skin. Humidifiers can replace a lot of missing moisture, and the simplest machine (available at Sears or your local hardware store) is usually the best. I like the type that you fill once a day, rather than those with large water reservoirs, which can be breeding grounds for germs. It's still important, though, to scrub the humidifiers out regularly with vinegar to keep them clean and bacteria-free. In a pinch, simply place a bowl of water on your heat source, filling it on a daily basis to make sure it keeps throwing humidity back into the room.

An ionizer is another good investment. These plug-in gizmos help absorb dust and pollution from the air, freshening the environment. Also, try to fill your home with plants; they pump out oxygen (just think of the difference in air quality when you walk in the woods or step into a park). Besides, it's glorious to have nature growing around you. Plants not only re-oxygenate the place but also help the humidity level as the water evaporates from the earth in the pot.

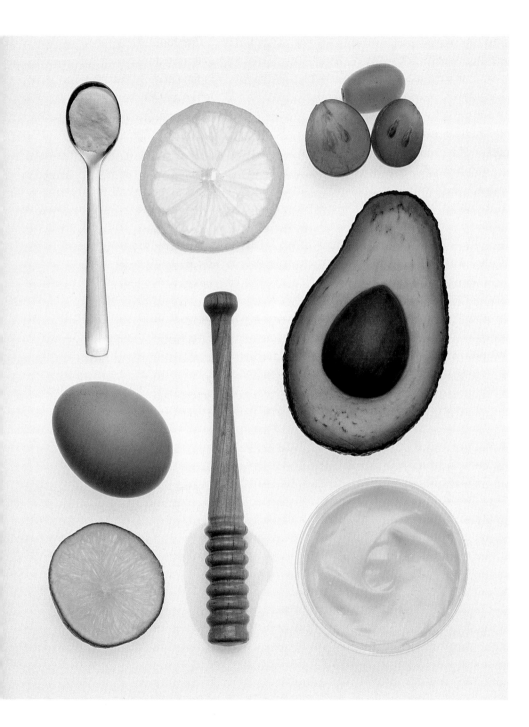

MY HONEY-AVOCADO TONING MASK FROM PHILIP B.

My friend Philip—creator of the wonderful Philip B. ("I-can't-do-without") hair products—created this rejuvenating honey-avocado mask for me to tone, cleanse, and tighten my skin. Philip assures me that the buttery flesh of the avocado, with its 20 percent fat content, penetrates aging skin and leaves it healthy and glowing. The grapes soften and moisturize the skin and the mayonnaise tones and smoothes. The baking soda provides deep cleansing action, gentle enough for even the most sensitive skin.

Botanical Formula

$1/2$ ripe avocado (peeled and pitted)
3   seedless green grapes
1   whole egg
1   teaspoon mayonnaise
1   teaspoon honey
1   teaspoon baking soda
1   teaspoon lemon extract
1   teaspoon lime extract

In a blender, puree the avocado, adding grapes one at a time. When smooth, add remaining ingredients and blend on medium speed for 45 seconds. This formula will not remain homogenous; mix well before each application. Apply evenly to face, and leave on for 10 to 15 minutes. Makes $1/2$ cup. Cover and refrigerate immediately. Discard after 3 days.

SKIN-CARE GLOSSARY

Here is the lowdown on some ingredients you might find listed on popular skin-care products and their literature:

AHAS (ALPHA-HYDROXY ACIDS) (citric, glycolic, lactic, malic, or tartaric): The role of AHAs in the anti-aging battle is to brighten the look of your skin rather than actually reduce the appearance of wrinkles. As chemical exfoliatiors, these acids loosen the flaky, dead layer of skin, improving skin texture and color and speeding its renewal. And, although AHAs exfoliate, they also trigger a thickening, bolstering process that boosts skin's moisture-holding properties and vital elastin fibers. Some women may experience irritation with the use of AHAs, so caution is advised.

ANTIOXIDANTS (vitamin E, a.k.a. tocopherol; vitamin C, a.k.a. ascorbic acid; beta-carotene): Some experts believe that antioxidants may turn out to be our most vital weapons in the fight against aging for their two-way approach in repairing skin and preventing further damage. Much of the environmental damage to our skin is the result of free-radical assault—from smoke, pollution, and UV rays. Free radicals turn the vital oils in the skin's surface rancid, damaging collagen, the protein fibers that serve as the building blocks of the skin. A growing number of products are being formulated with antioxidants, (especially vitamin C and vitamin E) to neutralize free radicals before they have a chance to ravage the skin. Some companies are developing even more potent free-radical fighters from land and sea botanicals. In the war against aging, antioxidant vitamins A, C, E, and beta-carotene play a vital role not only in your skin care, but also in your diet.

BETA-HYDROXY ACIDS
These are the close relations of AHAs, performing the same skin-brightening task. The best known beta-hydroxy compound is salicylic acid. However, as with AHAs, anyone experiencing irritation with them should discontinue use immediately.

CERAMIDES These lipids, found in the spaces between the skin's own cells, help stabilize the skin's structure by retaining moisture—so they're of great benefit to older, dry, or damaged skins.

COLLAGEN Collagen's ability to attract water to the skin makes it a superb moisturizing ingredient. Collagen applied to the surface of the skin in a cream, however, cannot rejuvenate the connective collagen in the skin (which is mainly responsible for firmness, or lack thereof).

ELASTIN Elastin is naturally present in your skin; it's what gives it the "bounce-back" factor (elastic = elastin). Elastin is also used as an ingredient in some moisturizers. While it can't actually repair the damage to your skin's elastin from the outside in, the large size of this protein molecule helps create a barrier on the skin, to seal in your skin's own moisture.

ENZYMES Enzymes—proteins derived from botanical ingredients like pineapple and papaya—can help even out your skin tone and texture. Enzymes are being touted as great new AHA alternatives since they encourage exfoliation with less irritation.

HUMECTANTS Humectants, including glycerine, sorbitol, squalene, and urea, attract moisture from the air to the surface of the skin. They are widely used in moisturizers, so there's little need to seek them out on their own.

MILK PROTEINS Milk proteins have been discovered to smooth, firm, and soften the skin. They can also be helpful in inhibiting irritation in skin.

OXYGEN boosts cellular activity and turnover, improving skin glow. The best way to deliver oxygen to your skin is a good brisk walk or another form of aerobic activity. Recently, oxygen has become a fashionable new ingredient in some moisturizers, but according to most skin-care experts, it's impossible to deliver oxygen to the skin via a cream. So keep on walking.

TEA (green tea, black tea): Tea contains polyphenolic acid, a powerful free radical scavenger (in other words, it's another antioxidant like vitamin A, C, and E). It's also very calming to the skin. Many experts are predicting that teas will have a growing impact in the field of anti-aging—in skin creams and as a health-boosting drink (see Vital Vitamins p. 137).

VITAMIN A (a.k.a. tretinoin), first turned up as an anti-acne treatment in the prescription product Retin-A. But when dermatologists—and patients—noticed that it was having a beneficial effect on patients' skin texture and wrinkles, they began to explore its other potential uses. Research showed that vitamin A encourages collagen production in the dermis, causing the middle layers to plump out and retain moisture more efficiently. Although Retin-A is still prescribed for cosmetic applications, newer vitamin A-based products (like Retinova from Ortho Pharmaceuticals) have been developed specifically for the treatment of premature aging of the skin. As with any prescription product, certain warnings are in order: Pregnant women are advised not to use tretinoin products and, since they have a thinning effect on the skin, exposure to the sun is forbidden. (You must religiously use a high-SPF sunblock; be sure to choose a sunblock that contains titanium dioxide rather than chemical sunscreens, which can trigger irritation). Less potent (and therefore less potentially problematic) derivatives of vitamin A, known as retinyls, are being incorporated into many anti-aging skin-care products and may also enhance skin radiance and smoothness.

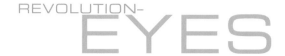

REVOLUTION-EYES

Our eyes not only let us see the world, they are what the world usually sees first when it looks at us. And, as we all know, first impressions are everything . . . so be sure your eyes attract, enhance, communicate—and sparkle!

The eye zone is the most delicate part of the face—and the area that registers age first. It's where laugh lines first start to appear, where gravity first tugs, and where our stresses, fears, and disappointments are revealed to the world. (Hands are the other giveaway.)

But think about it: Laugh lines communicate happiness. Crinkles around the eyes chronicle the joy in your life, of time spent in the delicious release of laughter. And, for that reason, I think we should simply learn to love and celebrate them. (They're a world away from those unflattering frown lines or unforgiving, deep forehead creases, which often reflect an unhappy soul.) And one thing is certain: Laugh lines certainly sound a lot more attractive than "crow's-feet," which is a term I think should be banned as of right now.

Because of its vulnerability, the eye area does need extra TLC on a dedicated, daily basis. The skin around the eyes has few oil glands of its own—and being thin and delicate, it can get papery. As a result, the skin around the edge of the eye should be patted with moisturizer regularly, using a cream that's designed for the special needs of this fragile area. (Many face creams are too rich or not gentle enough. Because moisturizers can "travel" into the eye, it's important to buy a product made especially for the eye area.)

Carry a little pot of eye cream in your handbag; during the day, regularly pat it around the corner of the eye. It not only counterbalances the drying effects of heating and air-conditioning, but it also imparts a slightly dewy appearance, a look that is younger and fresher than dry, parched skin. And of course, take special care to moisturize the eyes at night.

Sleeping at night in one position can literally "sleep" lines into your face. If you habitually sleep on just one side, you may notice that the creases, and eventually the lines and wrinkles, are worse on that side of your face, where it gets "smooshed up" by your pillow or your hand. It's hard to change the sleeping habits of a lifetime, but do try; if that area isn't continually scrunched at night by the way you sleep, those creases and resulting lines will relax and become less evident over time.

REAL-EYES SOLUTIONS Puffy eyes, alas, tend to be hereditary. But puffiness can also signal a reaction to what we're putting inside our bodies. Chinese, Japanese, and processed foods often contain MSG (monosodium glutamate), a flavor enhancer that can set off almost instantaneous water retention. So nowadays, I order MSG-free food; ask for the soy sauce with a green lid (which is low in sodium) and check labels in the grocery store. Alcohol and prescription drugs can also trigger puffiness. The alcohol may create damage under the eye and on the lid, abnormally swelling and creasing the skin. In addi-

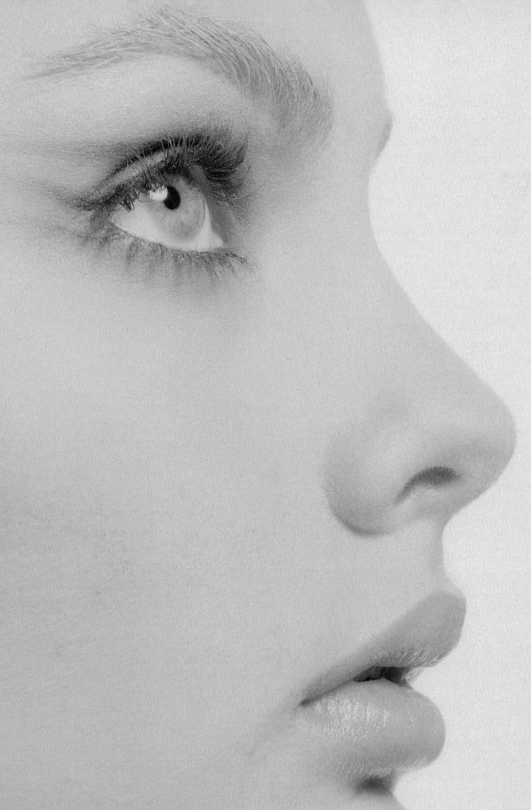

"IN YOUTH WE LEARN,
IN AGE WE UNDERSTAND"

SIMONE DE BEAUVOIR

tion, you should be aware that food allergies or sensitivities—even to everyday foods like wheat or dairy products—can set off the problem as well. So if you have a tendency for swelling under the eyes, check your eating and drinking pattern, and then make necessary lifestyle adjustments. You'll be amazed at how much control you can exert!

Let's face it: As we get older we tend to look a little better later in the morning. We do get there . . . but like many things at this age, it just takes a bit longer. So if you're prone to eye bags, my advice is to try to schedule those special moments a little later in the day and to make use of the following suggestions:

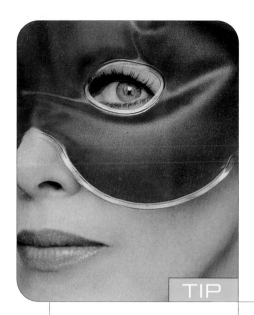

- Gently tapping the under-eye area can help drain away everyday or morning-after-the-night-before puffiness. Take your middle finger and very lightly pat under the eye, all along the cheekbone and up to the side of the temple. Repeat, repeat, repeat, backward and forward very softly.

- Soothe puffy eyes with a sesame-filled "bean bag," placing it on your eyes while lying down. These bags—usually covered in silk—weigh down the eyelid, relaxing the eye muscles and soothing the area (see Resources). I find this blissfully relaxing. It eases tension around the eyes, especially if you've been reading too much or working too long on the computer. Your eyes will feel revived just minutes after using the weighted bag.

- Cold milk. Pour ice-cold milk onto two cotton pads and place them on your eyes for ten minutes. In no time, the swelling will go down.

- Teabags can work wonders! Dip them in warm water, squeeze out the excess liquid, and place them on your closed eyes for ten minutes. This is great to do before an important event or as a quick eye-opener in the morning. (Tea bags are even more effective if you refrigerate them for 10 to 15 minutes before applying.)

Some women swear by those gel-filled "ice masks" that you keep in the icebox for "puffy eye" emergencies. (You can find them in most pharmacies.)

- Take a cold washcloth or a bag filled with ice chips and place it over the eyes—taking the opportunity to put your feet up and relax a little bit before a big event.

- Keep a jar of eye cream in the fridge (especially in summer). Smooth on the cold eye cream or gel to reduce swelling—just make sure it sets before you apply any makeup.

- There are eye gels available that remedy puffy eyes almost instantly. Lancômes's Bienfait and Clarins' Contour des Yeux are particularly good.

- To take the redness out of bloodshot eyes, I swear by Visine drops and a French product, called Colyre Blue, that many makeup artists use. It seems to make blue eyes bluer and the whites of eyes whiter. Also, avoid smoking and smoke-filled rooms, don't strain or overstress your eyes, and be sure to get plenty of sleep.

Finally, it never hurts to just lie down and take a rest—your eyes will reflect your refreshed energy and spirit. The better care you take of them, the brighter they'll sparkle.

A GLASS ACT Glasses are fun. They can dramatically change your personality in a second and make a terrific fashion statement. I love to do makeovers on friends, and often the first thing I suggest is trying out a new pair of glasses. I prefer to shop for my glasses with a friend—or with my daughter, who is never shy about telling me which styles are (and aren't) age appropriate. (We don't always agree!) A lot of the time, you can't really see how you look in glasses. A good tip, though, is to use a handheld mirror to look at your reflection in the larger looking glass. That second reflection is how other people actually see you, and may give you a better idea of how certain frames suit your face and personality.

You can use glasses strategically, for an instant change in the way you look and come across. Put Michelle Pfeiffer in a pair of glasses, for instance, and she looks much more serious. Put a pair on Julia Roberts, and she looks funky. Take off Sally Jessy Raphael's, and she loses her spunk! I like the idea of building a wardrobe of frames that reflect different dimensions of your personality. After all, your closet has your work attire, dressy dresses, and jeans, right? So, have fun, express yourself, and complement your look with glasses.

Older women, I've noticed, tend to wear very big glasses—which can look aging and old-fashioned on many of us (Jackie Kennedy and Audrey Hepburn were exceptions to the rule). I prefer a smaller frame, which is fresher looking, more modern, and youthful. (Check out the Paul Stuart line, which I've found is very flattering; you can find his frames at most retail eye stores.)

Sunglasses are also crucial. They not only protect your eyes against harmful UV rays, but the right shape can stop the sun from sneaking into the area around the eyes as well. Dark lenses and side arms also help to prevent squinting, so look for shapes with wide arms or wraparound frames that actually cover up the laugh-line area. These offer that "little-bit-more" protection, and in the age-prevention battle, every little bit counts.

I once attended an elegant dinner at Maxim's in Paris for Sharon Stone. She wore a floor-length blue gown, black gloves, and mysterious, blue-tinted sunglasses—which she did not take off the entire evening. She finally explained, "I just got off a plane and I'm just so tired." She was using the tinted glasses as makeup. She solved a problem by creating a unique fashion look that was fabulous!

Take time to choose. Experiment! Ask advice. Because glasses can add ten years if they're wrong—and take off five, if they're right.

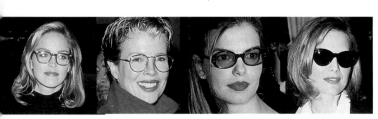

Sharon Stone   Kim Basinger   Jeanne Tripplehorn   Michelle Pfeiffer

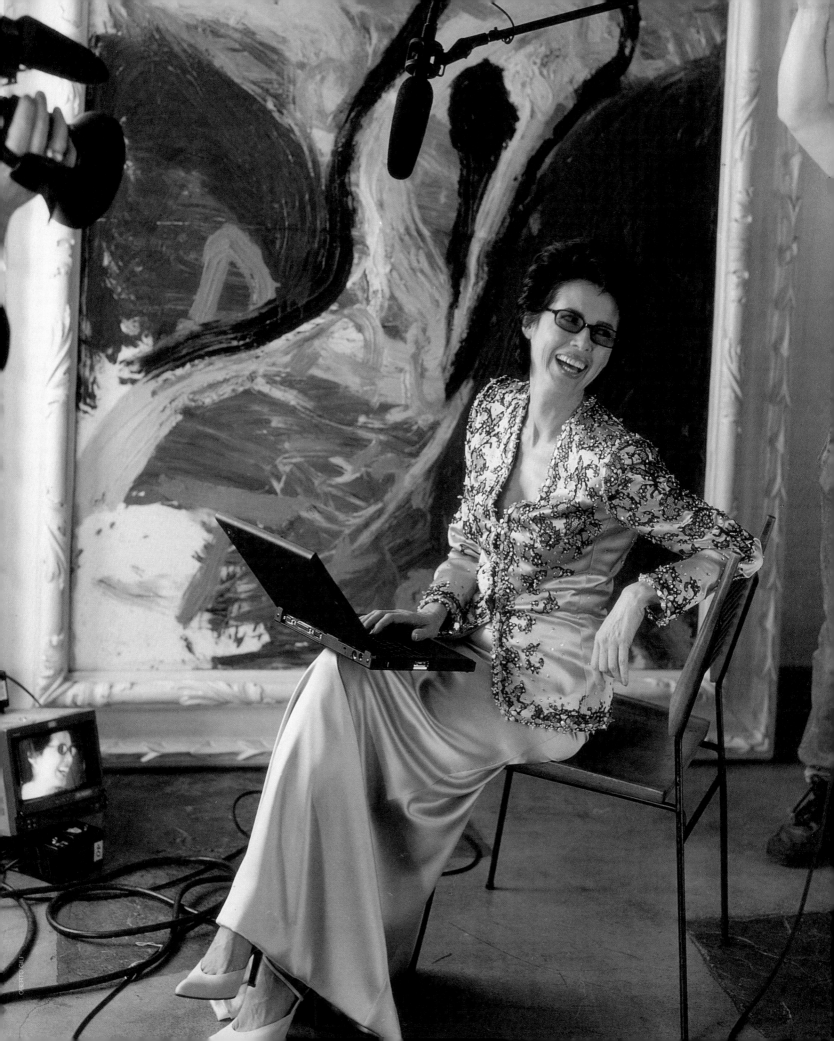

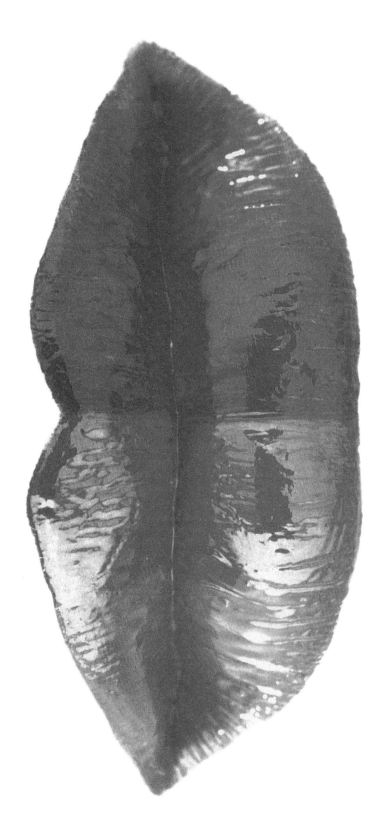

As we get older, our lips get thinner. They literally lose some of their fat, which is why, as we age, lips can become a real anxiety zone, even for women who've never been insecure about them before. What's more, the fragile skin around (and especially above) the lips is prone to fine lines, which often causes lipstick to bleed and feather. So as body parts go, our lips are one of the more vulnerable areas to the visible signs of aging.

The key is to nourish, nourish, nourish. The skin on the lips comprises only three to five layers of skin—compared to fifteen elsewhere on the body—so they tend to lose moisture quickly. If you keep your lips well-slicked with a balm, a cream, or a creamy lipstick, it actually creates a physical barrier that stops evaporation and prevents them from drying out. So, day and night, slather on the moisture. And, during daylight hours, add an extra element of UV protection, because lips are particularly vulnerable to sun damage (which speeds up the wrinkling process). In summer, especially, protect your lips with a high SPF—preferably 25 plus.

I'm a big fan of lip gloss for maintaining skin condition and giving the optical illusion of fuller lips. Kiehl's lip balm is one of the all-time greats to combat the effects of air-conditioning or heating. It's handy to keep on your desk or in your handbag . . . and don't forget to use it when you fly.

To keep your lips hydrated, you might try applying a really thick

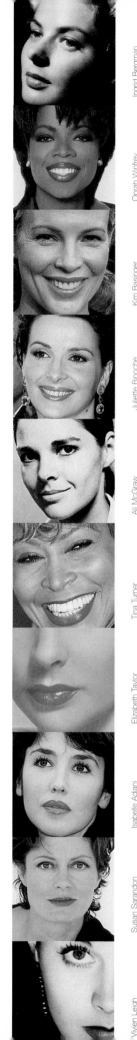

Ingrid Bergman

Oprah Winfrey

Kim Basinger

Juliette Binoche

Ali McGraw

Tina Turner

Elizabeth Taylor

Isabelle Adjani

Susan Sarandon

Vivien Leigh

layer of balm at night—almost like a "mask" for lips—and let it soak in. If they are chapped and sore, don't ever pick at the skin; it's painful and causes them to look worse. However, flakes of skin can look unattractive as well as make for patchy lipstick. There is a way to buff away the flakes of skin without causing harm to the lips:

1   Wet your lips with a compress (i.e. Kleenex, cotton, wool, or a flannel soaked in hot water).
2   Keep the compress pressed against your lips so that they absorb the moisture.
3   Use the fabric of the compress to lightly exfoliate your lips. Don't try and take off more skin than what comes away easily and naturally.

How can you avoid the feathering and bleeding that goes hand in hand with smoker's lip? Give it up . . . the smoking, that is. Constantly puckering while dragging on a cigarette is just begging for fan-like lines that attract lipstick like a magnet. And, with aging, they only get worse. If all of the other major health concerns don't inspire you to give up smoking, then maybe vanity will. In fact, it is never too late to reverse at least some of the damage. Give up the habit of puckering to smoke, and skin will become smoother again, in time.

Fuller lips are a common fantasy women have—perhaps because the lips are such a symbol of sensuality and sexuality; a physical reminder of the delicious possibility of intimacy! Lips we love—and long for—include Oprah's, Michelle Pfeiffer's and Kim Basinger's. Amazing makeup tricks can re-create that fullness very effectively, but for some women, plumping up lips with collagen or Gore-Tex (yes, the same fabric that's used for outdoor gear) is the solution to the problem of thinning lips.

A cosmetic surgery twofer is "autologous fat injections"; this procedure takes fat from elsewhere in your body and injects it into the lips. Don't forget, however, that over a period of a year, collagen and autologous fat both disappear back into the body—so ongoing treatments are needed to maintain your plumped-up look. Gore-Tex is a lifetime solution, but none of these procedures should be undertaken lightly and you should consult with a plastic surgeon or a cosmetic dermatologist to decide whether this procedure is for you. While full lips may be sexy now, looks change, so beware of permanent solutions simply for a trendy look.

Remember: You wouldn't want to be kissed by lips that are dry and scaly—nor does anyone else. Lips are an extremely sensitive area of the body. With correct care and nourishment, at any age, we can continue doing what soft, moist lips do best: to kiss, kiss, kiss — your children, your friend, your husband, or sweetheart.

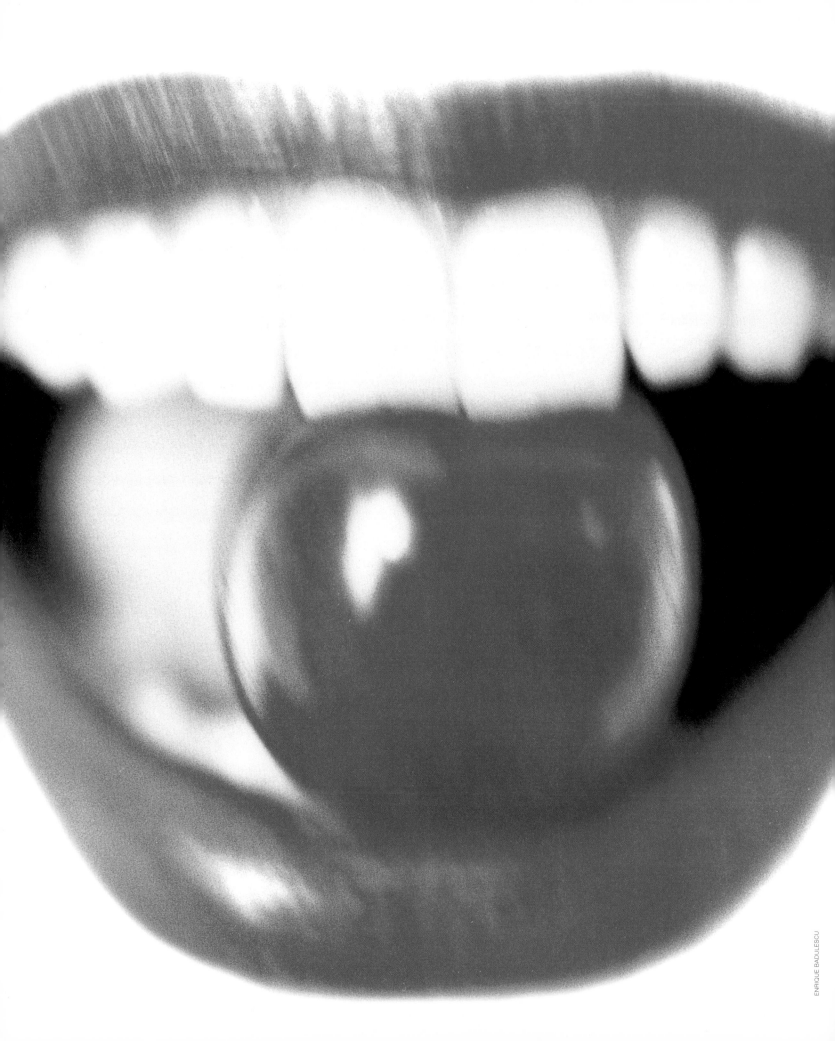

TEETH
THE SECRETS OF A DAZZLING SMILE

A smile instantly melts the heart and lifts years from your face. But if your teeth aren't looking their best, it can ruin your look and sap your confidence. Certainly, when it comes to teeth, we all want a stunning smile. Personally, I find myself riveted by someone's smile, especially when they have beautiful teeth. The strength of a great smile can dazzle and disarm; a smile is a wonderful "upper" and just makes us (and everyone around us) *feel* good.

As we age, teeth are more vulnerable to staining—from red wine, tea, coffee. For a few hours after drinking any of these, teeth can look dull and dingy or slightly brownish or bluish, and over time, these stains can become permanent. (If your teeth are prone to staining, steer clear of these drinks—and foods, like berries.) Brushing regularly, for a minimum of two minutes twice a day, is a must, but every four to six months you should get your teeth cleaned professionally as well. It's also good to change your toothbrush every three months, as by then it has lost its effectiveness and is prone to bacterial buildup.

At this stage in life, we should all be flossing with almost religious fervor. Particles of food stuck between teeth lead to killer breath and potential gum disease. Eating plenty of raw fruits and vegetables is a natural way to clean the teeth and stimulate the gums during the day, but only regular flossing removes the plaque debris from between teeth and around the gums. As we age, the gums recede and you can see more of the root of the teeth—a spot-it-at-ten-paces sign of aging. Also, the reason we lose teeth is generally because of our gums, not the teeth themselves.

KEEP YOUR BREATH SWEET
Bad breath is a big turnoff for all of us. The impact of a beautiful, well-dressed woman is ruined when you get close enough to discover she has bad breath; it screams "old." Carry breath mints or sprays on you at all times and floss between meals whenever possible. Try to keep a toothbrush handy between meals and also Stimu-Dent toothpicks, which massage the gums and help stimulate circulation.

For some people, bad breath is the result of a digestive problem or a sluggish elimination system. The breath is one of the ways the body excretes toxins. If you don't take care of your body—and watch what you eat—food can back up in your system. Walking, exercising, eating well, and drinking lots of water can help prevent constipation—and keep bad breath at bay. You might also want to try supplementing your diet with acidophilus (friendly bacteria that help re-balance the gut) or with digestive enzymes (from a company called Cell-Tech) which help improve digestion (see Resources).

Tongue scraping is another remedy for bad breath. A common practice in the East for hundreds of years, cleaning the tongue with a fine stainless steel scraper is a safe and effective way for removing bacteria that collects in the mouth (see Resources).

TIP

Become best friends with your dentist—regular cleanings are the most effective way to keep bad breath at bay. And that way, you'll have the confidence to keep smiling forever.

DESIGNER SMILES

The days of visiting the dentist purely to have a cavity filled or a quick polish are history; there are several fast fixes offering brighter, whiter teeth. The world of cosmetic dentistry has become seriously high tech, with new techniques to fix a less-than-perfect smile being perfected all the time. If you are self-conscious about your teeth, you might want to consider making an investment in your smile (see Resources).

BLEACHING

This is the simplest and least expensive way to great white teeth. Depending on the degree of discoloration and the number of teeth to be treated, in-office bleaching can take from one to six visits, with a minimum of a half hour on each tooth.

The most common "home bleaching" technique involves a plastic "tray," which is designed for your mouth by your dentist, filled with a hydrogen peroxide solution, and worn at night for a period of roughly two to three weeks. By penetrating the pores in the enamel, the solution bleaches out the discoloration.

In addition, there is a new laser-bleaching process, for bleach-resistant teeth. The gums are protected with beeswax before a solution of hydrogen peroxide is applied directly to teeth, which are then zapped with a blue-light laser, then a CO_2 laser. As a final step, teeth may be treated with a fluoride glaze, to improve shine and help resist future stains. But as with all bleaching/tooth-whitening procedures, upkeep is critical; you'll need to use a calcium peroxide toothpaste (like Supersmile or Colgate) to maintain the gleam.

APPROXIMATE COST: $250 to $700

NOTE: According to tests carried out at UCLA, be aware that the solutions used by dentists may weaken tooth enamel. Over-the-counter bleaching kits are now available, which should also be used with caution—and only your dentist can tell you if you're a good candidate.

COSMETIC CONTOURING

This can help protruding or crooked teeth without the expense, time, hassle, and embarrassment of wearing braces. Using fine diamond stones and sandpaper disks, the dentist changes the shape of a tooth—or creates an illusion of straightness. It's painless—and usually doesn't take more than one visit per tooth.

APPROXIMATE COST: $200 to $250

BONDING

An alternative to yesterday's crowns, bonding can be used to change a tooth's shape or to cover dark stains. First of all, the tooth is lightly etched to create a base for a material called composite resin, which is then applied over the tooth. Although bonding can hide many sins, know that it can also result in a more opaque and bulkier-looking tooth than nature gave you—and that bonds may be vulnerable to breaking, staining, sensitivity—and even cavities. Finally, bonding must be redone every two to five years.

APPROXIMATE COST: $300 to $500

LAMINATE VENEERS

Laminate veneers are now more popular than bonding or caps, and can be used to correct worn-down, crooked, chipped, gapped, or seriously stained teeth. During a two- to four-hour appointment, teeth are prepared as the dentist removes between 0.2 to 0.5 mm. of tooth enamel, using either acid, a drill or a hand tool. Thin, tailor-made veneers, made of plastic or porcelain, are then applied with a resin cement to fix them in place. A high-intensity light beam then bonds the veneer to the tooth in just sixty seconds. Plastic veneers are cheaper than porcelain, but not as strong or as lifelike; they may need frequent professional cleaning to keep them dazzling. Porcelain veneers have a natural color and translucency; no solvent can weaken the bond and only drilling will remove them; the lifetime of a porcelain veneer is regularly around eight to fifteen years.

APPROXIMATE COST: $900 to $1,500

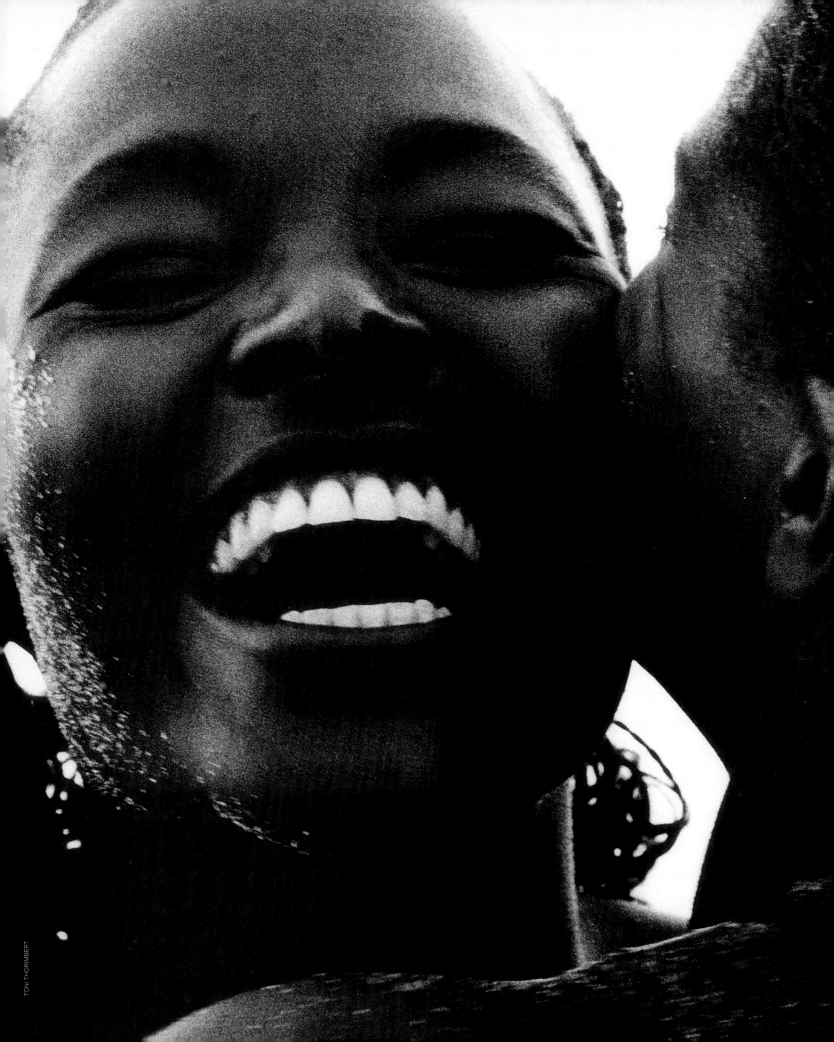

PROBLEM SPOTS & ANGST AREAS
AND LEARNING TO LOVE IMPERFECTION . . .

As we age, we develop problem spots—parts of our bodies that we are less than thrilled about. These areas of angst are basically a fact of life—usually caused by gravity over time, unhealthy eating habits, bad gene pool luck, lack of exercise, or the basic wear and tear of life. There are two ways to address problem spots and angst areas: work on changing them or change your attitude toward them. Probably, a balance of both is best.

Naturally, we'd probably all love to look the way we once did, but that just isn't realistic. At this age, I think it's so important to develop a deeper understanding and better acceptance of who we are now, rather than the constant worry about the appearance of a wrinkle, a pucker, or a droop. We've lived long enough to know that we are more than our dry skin, more than our wrinkles, more than our cellulite—or at least I hope so! Trust that the person you are now is worth the wrinkle or two you gained in the process. What we gain with age is well worth it . . . and well worth celebrating.

But there are some physical changes that we truly may find disturbing and that we don't necessarily need to endure. A few, such as age spots, dry skin, and increased facial hair, can be the result of hormonal changes. And luckily, some of these can be easily fixed—or at least prevented.

AGE SPOTS   Age spots, like freckles, are caused by sun exposure. They can appear on the cheeks, under eyes, and on the back of the hands. It is never too late to stop age spots from getting worse. The secret is to wear an SPF 15 or higher moisturizer on your hands and face, *every single day*. In addition, there are treatments to bleach out age spots: hydroquinone preparations or Retin-A, both prescription products that help to gradually return skin to its normal pigmentation. A last resort, because it's expensive, may be laser treatments, which must be carried out by a highly skilled medical professional experienced in this technique. No matter how you diminish or erase your age spots, you must continue to use sunscreen religiously or more spots will appear.

FRECKLES   (which I have and have learned to love!) Unlike age spots, freckles tend to appear in summer and fade somewhat in winter. Staying out of the sun can prevent their appearance, and eventually help them to fade. Don't try to completely cover up the ones you have with foundation or concealer, or you'll end up with a mask-like look.

DRY SKIN   Moisturize, moisturize, moisturize everywhere. As we age, oil production slows down, so we have to give nature a helping hand. Pay special attention to elbows, hands, heels, knees, and toes. Truly one of the all-time great

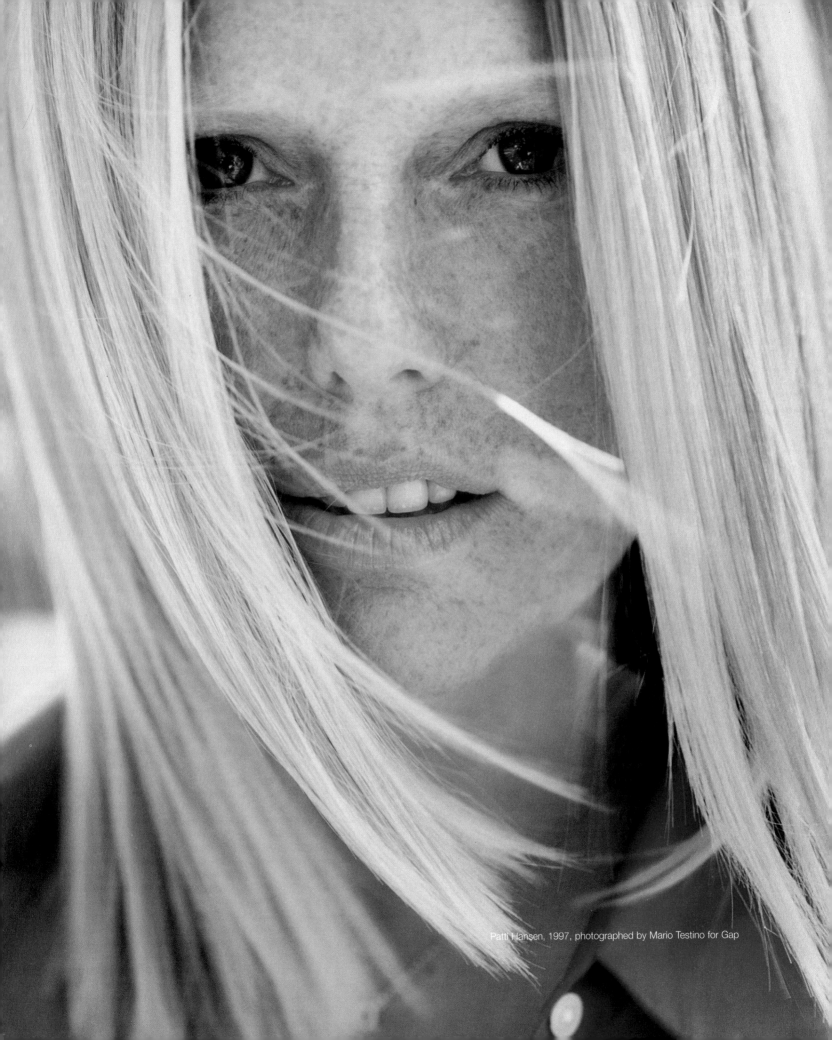

Patti Hansen, 1997, photographed by Mario Testino for Gap

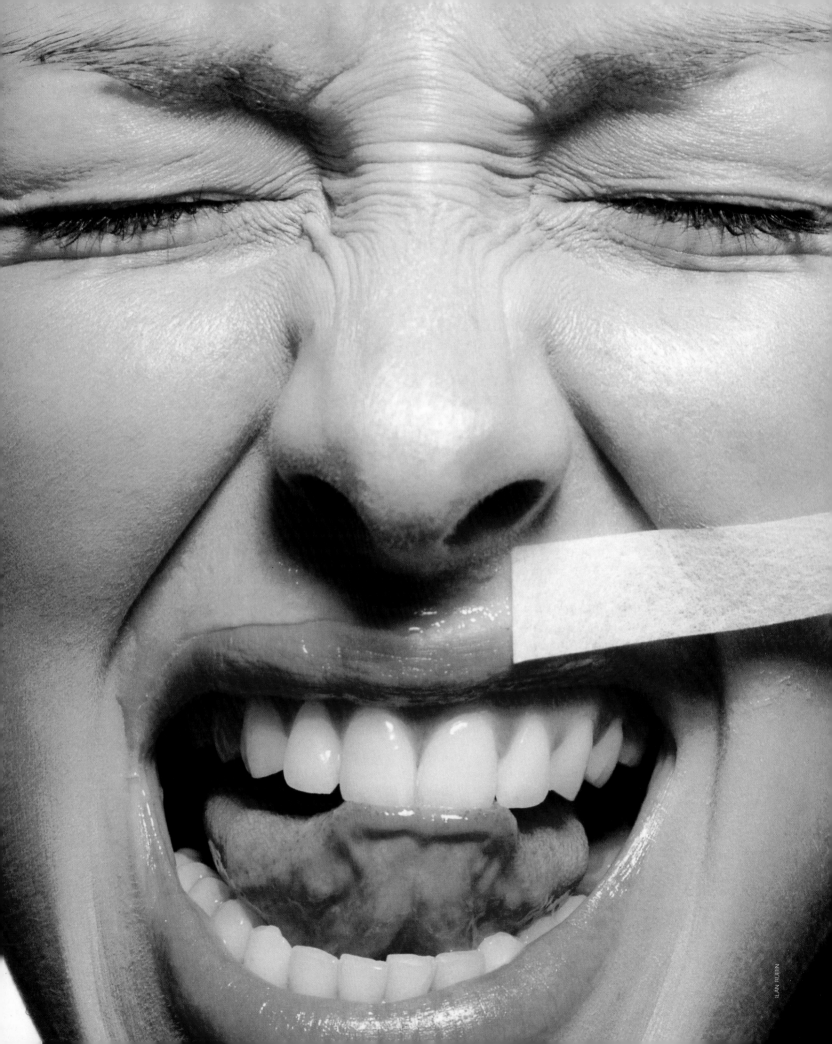

ILAN RUBIN

creams is Neutrogena Norwegian Formula Hand Cream. This is one of those products that beauty companies call "a sleeper." It started to take off when doctors, who wash their hands continually between patients, began using the rich cream to put back the moisture that anti-bacterial soaps were taking out. It is particularly effective in winter when hands are suffering the ravages of wind and central heating.

FACIAL HAIR   Be on the lookout for these annoying sprouts! Because at first glance, without a magnifying mirror and your glasses, you may not notice that there's a hair growing out of a mole or under your chin. Unfortunately, facial hair worsens with age. Don't snip or shave—you will end up with coarse regrowth. If there are only a few hairs, the simple solution is to pluck. If you have more general facial hair, there are several options you can try. One is bleaching. An inexpensive, easy-to-use bleach (such as Jolén) will make the hair less noticeable. If you feel the hair is still visible, try a depilatory cream (like Nair) that dissolves the hair just below the surface; the results last for around three weeks.

Alternatively, try "sugaring," a technique used since ancient Egyptian times; a sticky mixture of sugar and water is applied to the skin, then pulled off. (You can buy sugaring kits on the Home Shopping Network or have it done professionally.) Or try waxing, a similar technique that leaves skin silky-smooth; heated wax is applied to the skin with a wooden spatula and briskly yanked off after it hardens. Yes, like sugaring, it hurts and can leave your skin a bit irritated for several hours, but the results are great and last about six weeks. The disadvantage is that hair has to grow back a quarter of an inch before you can sugar or wax again, and you may not want to live with the interim stubble.

Two longer-term options are electrolysis, which uses a sterile needle and an electric current to permanently destroy the hair follicle, and laser hair removal, which is becoming more widely available. Be absolutely certain that your electrologist uses a new needle for each visit, and ask her to wear latex gloves to protect against infection. Laser hair removal was initially thought to offer a truly permanent solution, but as with electrolysis, some women find that hair does grow back over time. To find an electrologist in your area, contact the Guild of Professional Electrologists (see Resources).

MOLES   Everyone should see a dermatologist at least once a year to have her entire body checked for suspicious-looking moles; if you have a history of (or family history of) malignant melanoma, every three to six months. (Malignant melanoma, which is related to sun exposure, is a particularly deadly form of cancer and can strike at any age. But if it's caught early, it's highly treatable.) If you have any doubts about a mole, or if a mole bleeds, changes color, or changes shape in any way, see a doctor immediately. Ignoring warning signs can be fatal. Certain types of moles, called atypical nevi, can also be signals of increased risk for developing melanoma. Most moles, however, are natural and benign, but they will multiply with repeated sun exposure, causing your chest, neck, and arms to betray your age.

THREAD VEINS/SPIDER VEINS   These can appear on the legs—or on the face. Some women are particularly vulnerable to the patterning of blood vessels that resembles a spider's web. Spider veins tend to go hand in hand with a porcelain complexion, simply because they are more *visible* on light skin. Some experts believe that steering clear of spicy foods and extremes of temperature can minimize the risk of developing more veins, but in truth, the jury's still out.

There are, however, two fixes. Sclerotherapy involves a doctor inserting a tiny needle into the vein and injecting a saline solution. As the solution enters the vein, you can actually see the characteristic redness diminish before your eyes. Over a few weeks, the solution causes the vein to collapse and it disappears. The only problem is that some veins are too small for the needle to treat, and some are too large. Occasionally, treatment may trigger a skin ulcer or may simply fail to work. And there is always the possibility that new spider veins will appear and you may have to undergo future treatments.

Today, doctors are also using pulsed-dye lasers to remove facial thread veins on the nose and cheeks; these emit light waves, which are absorbed by hemoglobin molecules in the bloodstream. The hemoglobin is vaporized; this creates heat, which cauterizes the blood vessel wall. But be absolutely certain that the practitioner who treats your thread veins with a laser is experienced in the technique.

VARICOSE VEINS   If you walk regularly, eat a high-fiber, vegetable-rich diet, drink plenty of water, stay active, and maintain a healthy weight, you're well on your way to minimizing your chances of developing varicose veins. But what if you already have them (sometimes, women inherit a proclivity for them)? Some veins can be improved by sleeping with your feet raised; place blocks to elevate the end of your bed. Look for Lycra pantyhose—is there anyone out there who hasn't discovered the joys of Lycra? Lycra hose does almost as good a job as old-fashioned support hose, yet look terrific!

If your varicose veins are serious enough to need treatment, you have two options. Sclerotherapy (as for thread veins), entails injection of a solution into the vein itself, with no side effects, leaving little more than an invisible thread of scar tissue beneath the surface of the skin. (Treatment of large veins by sclerotherapy may mean that you have to wear compression stockings for several weeks afterward, and repeat treatments may be needed, depending on how many problem veins you have.) The resulting brown discoloration fades away within two years in over 90 percent of patients. If not, a copper vapor laser can be used to fully eradicate the marks. As with smaller problem veins, varicose veins may also reoccur, so maintain your good eating and exercise habits to best prevent new, unwanted veins.

Surgical stripping is the last resort in the treatment of varicose veins: the veins are actually removed from the legs through tiny incisions, with no impact on overall circulation. In some cases, all that's needed is a local anesthetic, which means an outpatient visit, although light general anesthesia is more common. You'll have to wear compression stockings for about six weeks afterward.

NIPS&
TUCKS

Cosmetic surgery is a personal decision. Only you can—and only you *should*—decide whether this is the right option for you; not a partner, not a friend, not a surgeon. I think there is a tremendous amount of pressure on women, as we age, to look younger than we really are, and this pressure can get out of control. Cosmetic surgery might seem like the magic answer. But shifting your attitude might be as effective (and is certainly cheaper) than adjusting your face or body parts. So try to re-evaluate what growing old really means. Personally, I believe that wrinkles and a little sagging are a small price to pay for the wisdom, experience, and confidence we gain over the years.

I would also suggest that before you rush to the more extreme step of cosmetic surgery, you try alternative approaches—skin care, self-care, exercise, and diet. These are the ministeps you can take before attempting a giant leap into the world of the knife and the laser. We certainly shouldn't be under the illusion that cosmetic surgery is going to fix our lives. Many women I have talked with find that once they've gone down the surgery route, it's often a slippery slope, leading to one round of surgery after another. But at the age we are, making adjustments with surgery is a personal decision. We definitely want to look the best we can, but just as importantly, we should be gently shifting the focus to an inner life.

If, after true soul searching, you decide that you really do want to opt for cosmetic surgery, you need to be armed with a substantial amount of information. This is elective surgery—not something to be undertaken lightly; it usually involves a general anesthetic, with all the associated risks (see suggested reading list).

These are just *some* of the solutions to some of the problem spots and angst areas. No matter what kind of physical imperfection you might think you have, what I believe is important at this stage in life is to shift our focus from the negative to accentuate the positive. So let go of the idea of those chubby knees, the panic about that new wrinkle, the horror of an extra pound—all those weak spots every woman feels are screaming and jostling for importance in her life. Change that channel and turn up the volume to: Yes! But what about those long, long eyelashes, that silky shining hair, dazzling smile, and manicured nails. Let *these* voices take over. Let's learn to accept (and maybe even love) our imperfections and focus on what's fabulous! There's a great big world out there—there's lots to do and it's all waiting for us.

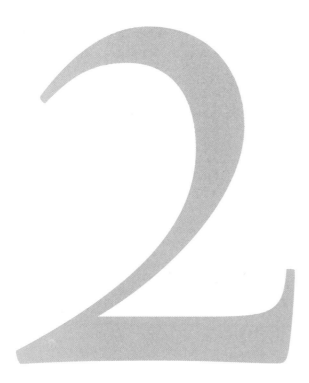

FABULOUS FACE-MAKING

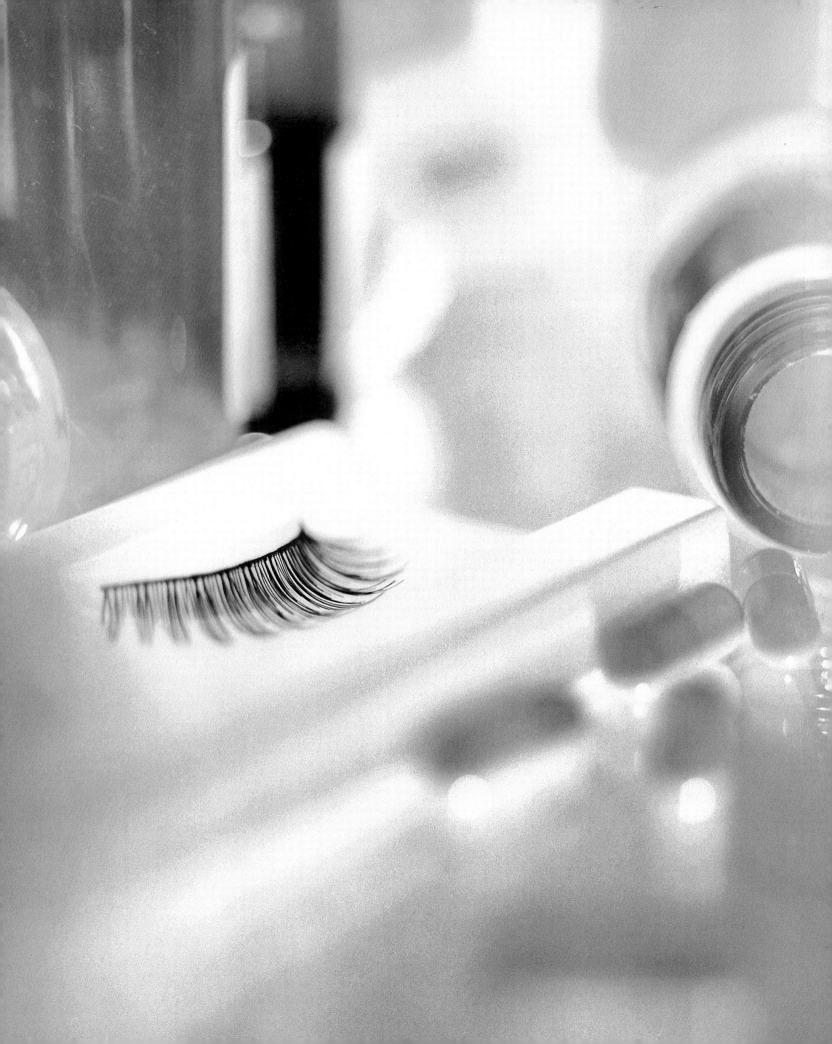

DAYLE'S MAKEUP SECRETS

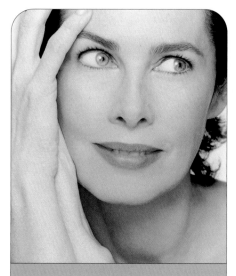

. . . to learn how to make the most of the face we've been blessed with. Working with the world's top professionals, I've learned that makeup can help us achieve the almost impossible: Put back the glow, take away the tiredness, even turn back the clock. With a few simple brushstrokes, you can erase years—and defy time. So let me share with you how to wave a magic (mascara) wand. Because making up— at any age—doesn't have to be hard to do.

Here are some of the secrets, tips, and tricks I've learned in thirty years of modeling and making films—because the right makeup can really turn back the clock.

FOUNDATION The old-fashioned way to test foundation color was on the back of your hand. Unfortunately, the color of that area usually bears no resemblance to your face tone. Surprised? Well, just put your hand next to your neck or jawline and see what a difference there is in tone. For color selection, just apply foundation along the jawline—one color on one side of your face, another shade on the other. Now, grab a hand mirror and check it in natural daylight (fluorescent light is totally misleading, so the lighting in a department store is usually the worst place in which to choose foundation). The right shade for you should disappear into your skin. But hands are still great to help you gauge coverage. By using the back of your hand you see how well a formulation blends in and covers veins and tone irregularities.

One of the big mistakes women make is choosing a base that's too pink. Aim for a color that matches your own skin color and disappears into your jawline and neck. Estée Lauder's Enlighten works wonders.

I like a moisturizing foundation with an SPF of at least 15, for extra sun protection. (As mentioned earlier, if you instead choose to apply foundation immediately after moisturizing or applying an SPF, it can make for a blotchy finish, so wait until the moisturizer has been fully absorbed before applying your base.)

Less is definitely more when it comes to foundation—especially as we age. I like my base to cover just the areas where extra help is needed—broken veins, under-eye shadows, the central T-area. I blend carefully in these spots, leaving the sides of my face makeup-free, which prevents the foundation from looking like a mask. (There's nothing more aging than a mask, especially if it's cracking.) You want your face to look and feel like natural, healthy skin.

With the right foundation, you may not need concealer. Avoid stick concealers, which can dry up and cake on the skin. Personally, I get the extra coverage I need from applying a second layer of foundation only where it's needed, dabbing it very gently on the skin with my ring finger. (The inner corner of the eye—where there are usually gray shadows—is a prime site for this; don't overlook it.) You can also use the layered foundation technique to cover up any age spots or veins. If you really want to be specific, use a small eyeliner brush lightly dipped in your foundation, then blend by pressing it gently into the area you want to cover. The heat of your finger will do the blending perfectly.

But at times, you may need the extra coverage of a concealer to even out skin tone and cover dark circles. My friend Regina, a beauty industry expert, vows she can't live without her "coterie of concealers"! Instead of foundation, Regina, at top speed, covers all the spots that count—under eyes, around the nose, by the mouth, and any blemishes. Her favorites she swears by: Trish McEvoy Protective Shield (#1) and Smash Box Foundation Stick (in "smashing beige"). The best ones I've found are Yves Saint Laurent's Touche Eclat (which comes with its own brush), and Lancôme MaquiComplet.

The same foundation shade probably won't work for you year-round— even if you do your damnedest to stay out of the sun. Sometimes, I take my lighter winter base and mix it with my summer one in the palm of my hand, using a finger to blend both shades; this way I can control the color and the level of coverage. It's a perfect technique for the seasonal changeovers—spring and autumn.

POWDER This is tricky, tricky, tricky—until you know how. It's a real danger area because too much powder (especially under the eyes) can have a seriously aging effect—it can cake, crack, and crumble. If you don't like to shine, then simply dab a little powder down the center of your face. I like to powder the inner part of the eye, the nose, around the mouth, and just a dab on the forehead. You have to be ultracareful not to powder the cheeks from the middle of the eyes outward toward the hairline; the powder will settle into the wrinkles under the eyes and emphasize them.

My favorite powder is Christian Dior's Plus Q'Invisible—an ultrafine pressed powder. I don't like loose powder as much because I feel it emphasizes the fine lines and wrinkles, especially those around the eyes. (I'm always telling makeup artists: "Hold the loose powder!" They're so used to making up eighteen-year-olds, they tend to load it on). You want to keep the powder as sheer and fine as possible. (Japanese rice powder can work well, too—Shu Uemura makes a great one, (see Resources). You can whisk this on with a small brush, which is easier to control than a big fat powder brush.)

I generally like a matte look. The only exception is for a fun night out, when a sexy light glow on the cheekbones and browbones can be attractive . . . and sometimes even on the collarbones and shoulders for all-over glimmer. FACE Stockholm makes a great cream shimmer named Radiance, which I find adds the perfect subtle glow to the face (see Resources). Choose a translucent, clear powder—nothing with color. All your powder is there to do is blot any shine, because you should be getting the color you need from your base and your blush.

If you have a tendency to shine, rather than applying layer after layer of powder, try old-fashioned paper blotters, which reduce the gleam; or try Estée Lauder Oil-Control Blotting Papers. You might also want to keep the glow at bay by applying Lancôme's wonderful T.CONTRÔLE gel to areas that are prone to oiliness. Just pat it on. It's great for camera work or if you're going to be somewhere really hot and need some control.

TIP

In summer, you might want to trade your foundation for a tinted moisturizer — one that gives just a little coverage. I love L'Oréal's Invisible Perfection (the shade I like is Opale), which has silicone particles that glide over the skin. It's a little more than a tinted moisturizer, a little less than a heavy base. It blends right in and becomes just like your skin—which is the whole idea!

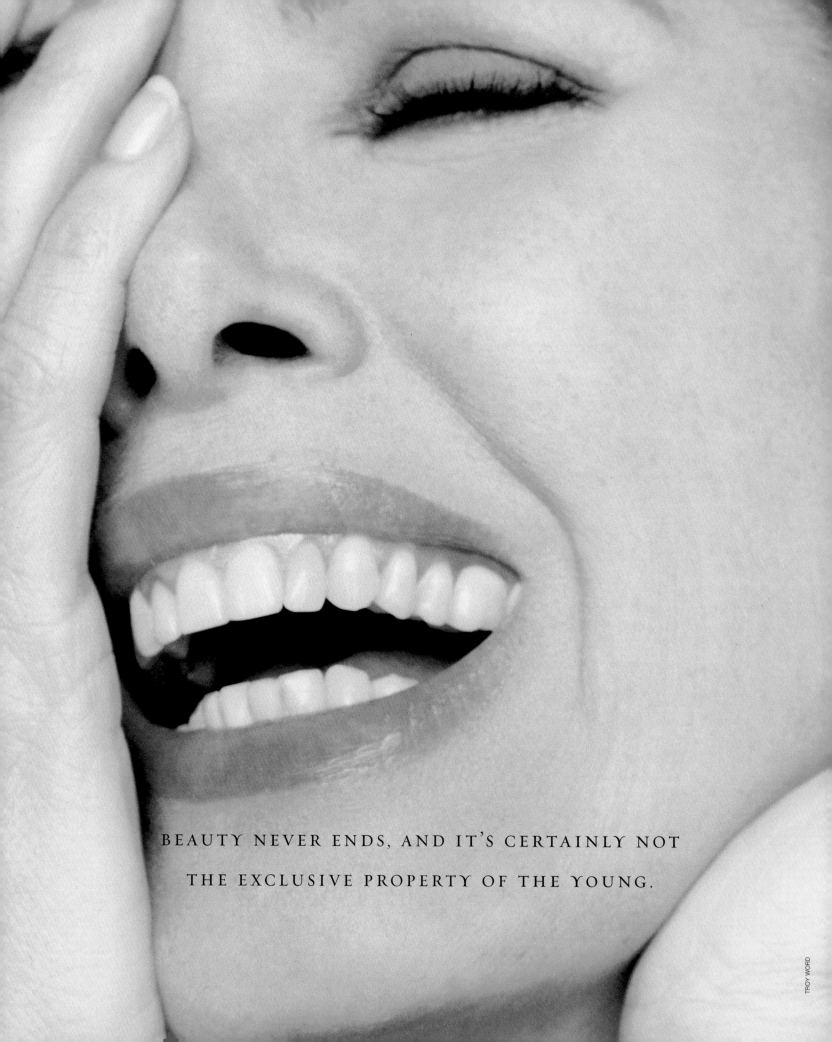

BEAUTY NEVER ENDS, AND IT'S CERTAINLY NOT
THE EXCLUSIVE PROPERTY OF THE YOUNG.

In summer, I apply a little terra-cotta powder, which gives a natural color while it absorbs the shine. I whisk it where the sun might naturally strike my face—around the hairline, on the nose and cheekbones plus the lightest touch on my eyes, for a hint of healthy color.

BLUSHER   During all my travels to different cities around the world, one of the most common beauty mistakes I see is the application of blush. Yet, applied perfectly, blush can take off years and restore the natural glow—even when we're feeling fatigued. The glow of a little cheek color gives a sense of health and youth. Just look at children with their rosy cheeks. That natural look is what we're trying to achieve.

It's crucial that the skin underneath the foundation is well-moisturized. That way any color added goes on evenly and stays on. The cheek color you choose should echo the color that you blush naturally. For me, blush color choice depends on the skin color I have at the time of year and the mood I'm in. If it's the middle of winter and I'm pale, I might brush on a soft pinkish tone, just to "lift" my face out of the doldrums. I wouldn't put anything on my skin that was too dark, because the contrast of blush color and my skin looks much too contrived. Remember: You want to suggest health by a tint instead of a swash of color. When your skin has more color in the summer, you can experiment with a deeper brown or bronze blush—but still, be sure to stay close to your own natural skin tone.

The blusher you choose for day won't necessarily be the one you wear for evening. Daytime calls for more natural shades: beiges and pinks. In the evening, try a stronger blush, taking your cue from the shade of lipstick you are wearing. The blush should come from the same color family as the lipstick: for example, pink with pinks, not orange or coral. A trick I often use: After applying my lipstick, I will rub my forefinger over the lipstick and gently "tap" the lipstick color ultralightly over my cheekbone, starting in a small circle and gradually working upward near the eye. Surprise! It is an instant rejuvenator. This also gives me the same hue on the cheeks as on the lips, and looks healthy, glowing, and natural—especially in summer, when you don't want to use as much powder.

So often I'm asked: Where does blush go? The answer is easy: Look in a mirror and smile (something you should be doing on a regular basis anyway)! The part of the cheek we call the apple is the fleshy part, right on the cheekbone. This is the area that should be blushed. (Don't stray too low—it makes the face look heavy in the jaw area.) Take a soft, medium-sized blusher brush and swirl it into the powder. Tap off the excess particles. On a smiling face, gently apply the blush in a circular motion on that "apple" (think high and up), gradually making the circles larger. Be very careful not to have any harsh edges; you shouldn't be able to see where the color starts and stops, so use the brush to blend, blend, blend. NOTE: Let me say again that a light touch is everything, especially with older skin. You want to treat your face with TLC at all times and avoid tugging on it. The final step is to lightly dust over the entire blushed area again with translucent powder. The result: a new, healthier, younger-looking you . . . in an instant!

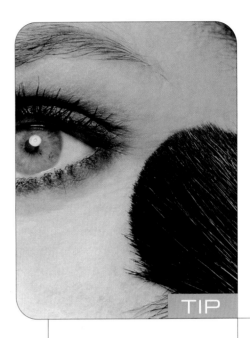

TIP

Another age-defying trick: when I'm really tired, I will sweep my blusher with the edge of a blusher brush slightly up from my cheek, toward the outside corner of my eye. It's like having an instant facelift. *Note: The brush head shouldn't be too fat and fluffy so that application is easier to control.*

One of the big mistakes women make is to end up with "skunk stripes": that dark wedge of color that runs along the cheek in a strip. This is the most common "blush error" that women make. Think about it: We don't blush in a stripe! It can be avoided by using those circular movements, rather than stroking blusher outward along the cheekbone. Do a double check: In your bathroom, you should have two mirrors, a hand mirror reflecting into the main mirror, enabling you to view your face from the side on. If there are any visible blush edges, take a cotton pad and gently "polish" the edges till they blend in.

The cream-versus-powder blush debate: Which one is best? I'm a fan of cream blushers for older skin: they contain moisturizing elements and avoid any hint of a "dusty" look, which tends to accentuate wrinkles. I like Francois Nars The Multiple—a gleam stick (see Resources)—to slick all over the cheekbone; also FACE Stockholm Radiance—great for evening glow. (All originally recommended by my daughter Ryan. Who says you can't share secrets between generations?) Cream blush should always be applied to a well-moisturized cheek, and it is a terrific option on days when you're not planning to wear foundation, enabling you to achieve an ultranatural look. Again, apply with gentle, circular movements, blending very carefully; working with the heat of your finger, dab, rather than stroke, the blush on. With cream blush, as with foundations and moisturizers, allow the natural warmth from your finger to heat up the product so that it glides on more smoothly and gently.

Powdered blushes can do the trick as well. I find you just have to pick a color and texture that leaves only a light veil of color on the skin, so you can control the intensity.

BROWS   Great brows frame the face beautifully. I never used to tweeze my brows. Actually, that was part of my trademark as a model, but I've noticed that as we get older, thinning the brows is a great cheat. It's like an instant eye lift. The eyelid skin tends to sag as we age, but the right brow shape immediately opens up the eye and disguises this.

You don't want to make brows pencil-thin, but you do want to groom them a little. And always think "up" as you work—tweeze them into an arch, from underneath, so that it gives the optical illusion of lifting your eyes. Changing your brow shape in this way can take years off. It's the quickest and most dramatic way to change your face, and it also gives a more finished look.

Do not even attempt to tweeze without a magnifying mirror and great tweezers—preferably Tweezerman (the makeup artists' tweezer of choice; see Resources); they make a slanted version for everyday use, and a "pointed" version for advanced users. You need the magnifying mirror because, without it, it's too easy to accidentally pinch the skin, and it also helps you to spot hairs that you'd otherwise miss. Try to tweeze away the blonde, fuzzy hairs, too, for a cleaner look—they pick up powder, otherwise.

You want to avoid having the outer part of your brows sloping downward toward your jaw. This downward slope of the brow only emphasizes the natural droop that happens as we get older. We want to counterbalance this tendency by thinking "up" again—tweezing and shaping to avoid that downward curve.

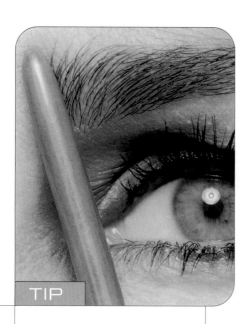

TIP

Your brows should start directly above the inner corner of your eye—line a pencil or a brush up with that, pointing straight upward, and tweeze anything that falls outside this line, between the brows. (Do not tweeze inside this line; it makes the space between the eyebrows too wide—it looks unnatural and detracts from the eye.)

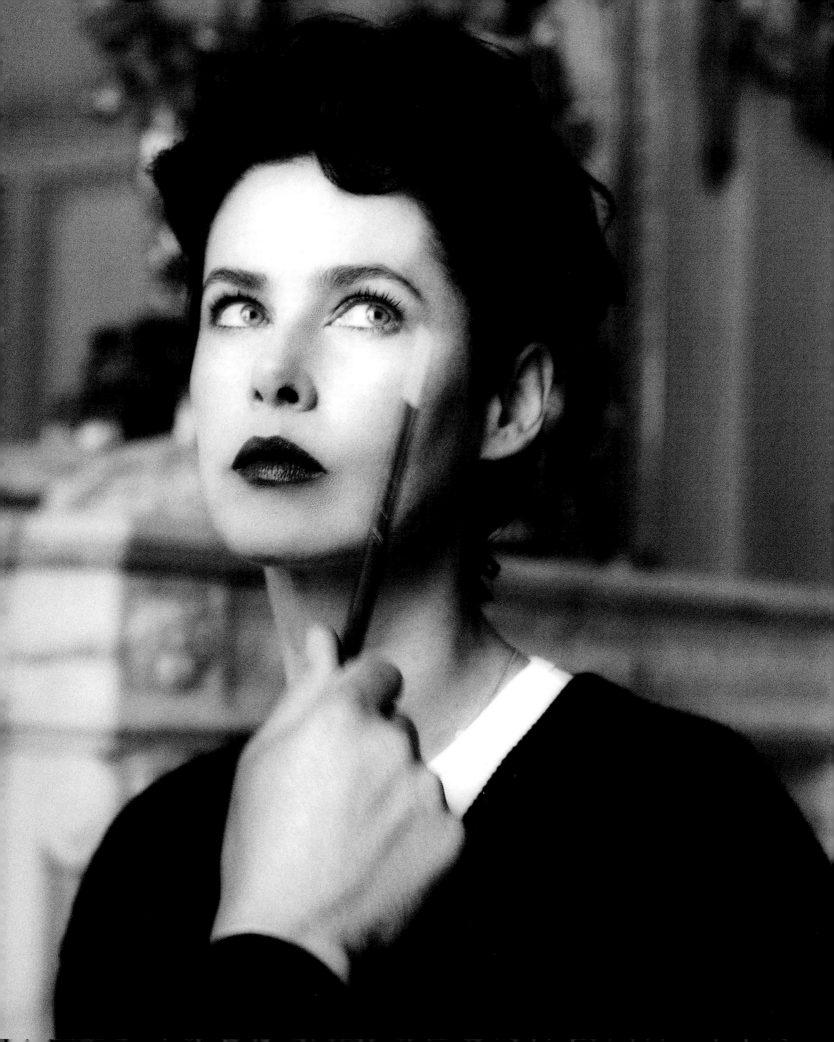

If you're nervous about tweezing brows into a new shape, experiment by lightly drawing in the new shape with a soft eyebrow pencil, so that you can try out a few looks.

As we age, our brows also thin. (If you've overplucked in the past, you may have patchy brows as well.) So I like to use a brown eyeshadow powder—in my case, dark brown—and an angled, thin brush to fill brows in. (I prefer powder shadow to pencil because it gives me more control and looks more natural.) Load on the shadow, then tap the handle brush on the edge of the sink to knock off any excess. Color from more or less the middle of the brow outward; if you put too much color on the inner corner, it can become too hard looking and appear as if you're frowning. Remember, you're trying to get the color onto the hairs themselves—not so much onto the skin, where the effect might be too obvious.

Gray-haired women can use a light gray color or taupey gray powder to color brows. Blondes can use paler taupe shades—but avoid anything with even a hint of rust or red in it. (Personally, I think blondes look fabulous with dark brows. Think of Sharon Stone—how strikingly her dark brows contrast with her blonde hair. Experiment!)

If you emphasize the hairs at the top of the brow, rather than the bottom, it contributes to that uplifted effect, too. (It's all an illusion—but who cares? This was a trick that Audrey Hepburn used.) After you've finished coloring your brows with powder, take your finger or a brush and groom them upward. A toothbrush or a child's toothbrush is also a great tool. You might want to look out for a special eyebrow gel (I like Tweezerman Brow Mousse), or a clear mascara like Cover Girl Natural Lash or The Body Shop Clear Mascara, which keeps brows groomed in place. Some makeup artists actually use hair spray lightly sprayed onto an eyebrow brush, then they stroke the brows in the direction they want. Because I have dark hair, sometimes after I've mascaraed my lashes, I take the wand with the leftover mascara and groom my brows upward, with little, tiny, feathery strokes. Whenever you're doing the brow area, your watchwords are lightly, lightly, lightly and up, up, up.

EYES

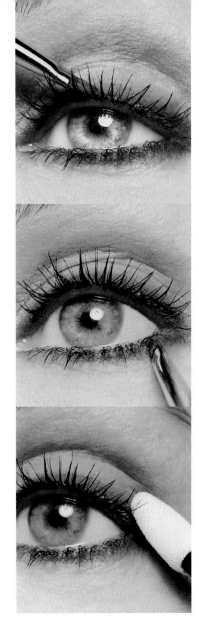

EYE LINING   To line the eyes, I take my skinny little eye-lining brush, wet it with water, and dip it into my darker brown shadow. I used to use a liquid liner, but I found that as I get older, liquid liner gives too harsh a line.

The trick for perfect eye lining is to look down into your mirror so that you can see the whole eyelid, revealing exactly what you're doing. (Practice really makes perfect here; you can rest your elbow on the table if you're less-than-steady handed).

1   Line the top and bottom of the eye, but on the lower lid, never go farther toward the nose than halfway.
2   Lift the line very slightly as you reach the outer corner of the eye.
3   Take the edge of your finger or a Q-Tip and smudge the line very slightly.

Lining the eyes like this gives the impression of really thick lashes—which is what we all long for.

SHADOW   The skin around the eye is the first area where aging starts to show. At a certain point, eye skin starts to droop and upper lids may become "hooded." You want to counteract this unfortunate fact of life with a clever use of powder. Use your magnifying mirror for these steps.

1   Start with your small, flat eyeshadow brush (Shu Uemura's No. 10 brush or Laura Mercier eyeliner brush is perfect for this) and a medium-brown shadow. From the center of the lowered lid, work outward and slightly upward, tracing the eye line along and close to the lashes.
2   Using a medium-brown shadow and an eyeshadow brush—again, Shu Uemura's No. 10 is perfect—shade the socket above the eye, always working from the outer edge inward. Direction is very important: if you work from the inside outward, you will inevitably take the line downward, in a curve, at the outer corner of the eye—which only emphasizes droopiness.
3   Once you've shaded, keep whisking with the brush until there are no obvious lines and the upper and lower shadow meet. You can also use your finger to smudge it. This technique works best for evening when the subtle lighting helps the results look natural.
4   With a smaller brush (which gives you more control), apply the brown shadow under the eye—close to the lash only as far inwards as the middle of the eye (taking the shadow all the way to the edge of the eye makes the eye look smaller).

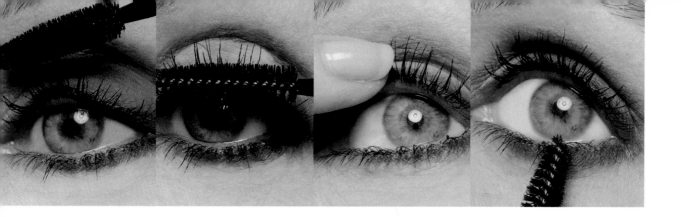

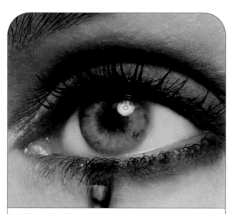

TIP

When I've finished my eye make-up, sometimes I'll take my blusher brush with the very last traces of blusher on (don't reload) — and whisk it over the eye area. This brightens and "lifts" the entire face and helps blend in the makeup.

DISGUISE PUFFY EYES

As discussed in the previous chapter, women develop a natural puffiness or pouchiness on the lower lid, just under the lash. Brown shadow will help disguise swollen eyes: the darker colors makes them appear to recede. Using a fine brush, lightly feather the powder along the puffy area just under the lash . . . and voilá! You have thicker lashes.

LASHES   Curling your lashes can make an eye-opening difference, but a lot of eyelash curlers can be pretty scary to use. It's so easy to catch your skin with them as you squeeze. However, there's a new patented little eyelash-curling gizmo by Ilise Harris (see Resources), which gives you much more control.

SIX STEPS TO PERFECT LASHES

1   Lightly wipe mascara wand on a Kleenex before using it on lashes; it gets rid of any excess blobs that end up clumping the lashes together.
2   Apply mascara on top of the lash first, rolling up from root to tip. This coats the lash so the wand has something to grip onto when applying mascara to the underside of the lash.
3   Then working from underneath, take the mascara wand and roll the lashes upward, almost pushing them into a curl.
4   Use your finger like a manual eyelash curler to push the lashes upward again. This curls and directs the lashes where you want them to go, making them look longer and opening up the eye.
5   When most of the mascara is off the wand and on the top lashes, move to the bottom lashes without dipping into the mascara tube again; this way, you'll avoid clumpiness (which is a common problem for older women— perhaps because we can't see as well when we're applying makeup). Don't wait for mascara to dry between coats; that also leads to clumpiness.
6   Holding the mascara wand vertically, zigzag it from side to side along the bottom lashes. If there are any clumps or blobs, use the mascara wand to stroke them away and separate each lash, so that the lashes are always pointing in the direction they naturally grow. (If you're steady handed, use a metal or plastic eyelash comb to separate and "de-clump.")

LIPS

Most women think their lips aren't full enough—and they're probably right. And unfortunately, as we age, our lips do get thinner. But what we don't want to do—ever—is pencil our lip line back where it used to be. When it comes to makeup, you're always going for subtlety and enhanced naturalness. So instead, pick a nude-colored lip pencil; two classics, which makeup artists favor, are Clinique's Raisin and Nars Morocco.

Applying lip pencil around your lips gives a more even edge and prevents lipstick bleeding into the feathery lines that arrive as we age.

1   Outline your natural lip line, using small, feathery strokes. You want to draw on the lip edge itself, emphasizing the natural line only by a fraction, with the lip pencil.
NOTE: If you've never done this before, complete only one side—either the upper lip or lower lip—and check out the results. Remember, you don't want the line to look obvious—just subtly enhanced. (Make absolutely sure that at the corners of the lips, the drawn line meets your own perfectly—to avoid the "clown" effect.)

2   To make the line look absolutely natural, take your first finger and gently trace the edge of the drawn lip line, so the heat of your finger softens the line, smudging it slightly so that it becomes almost invisible.

LIP COLOR   Try not to get stuck in a color rut with lipstick. (Blondes, particularly, seem to get hooked on reds.) If you look great in red, then terrific, but experiment to see whether there's a more flattering shade for you out there. My friend Michele was addicted to red lipsticks until I introduced her to browner, warmer, shinier shades—a newer, sexy look with her blonde hair and light skin. She saves red for big evenings. I just weaned my mother off red and onto browner shades, too. And I did an instant, sidewalk makeover on my friend Rusty as we were rushing to a meeting, transforming her too bright berry-red look to soft, glossy mauvey-brown lips, which she loved. So keep up-to-date with what's happening on the beauty pages of magazines; it doesn't mean you have to follow the trends slavishly, but they might inspire you to update your look and have fun with your face.

TIP

Throw out your mascara every three months. Old mascaras can be a breeding ground for germs, potentially triggering eye infections.

TIP

As a guideline, use any lip color that is just a shade darker than your natural, naked lip color — unless you are wearing reds, then the pencil should be as close to your lipstick color as possible.

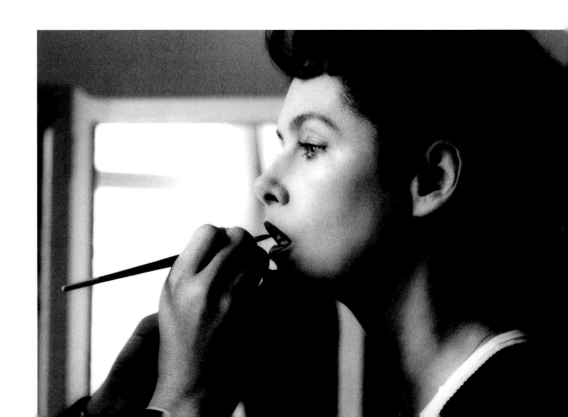

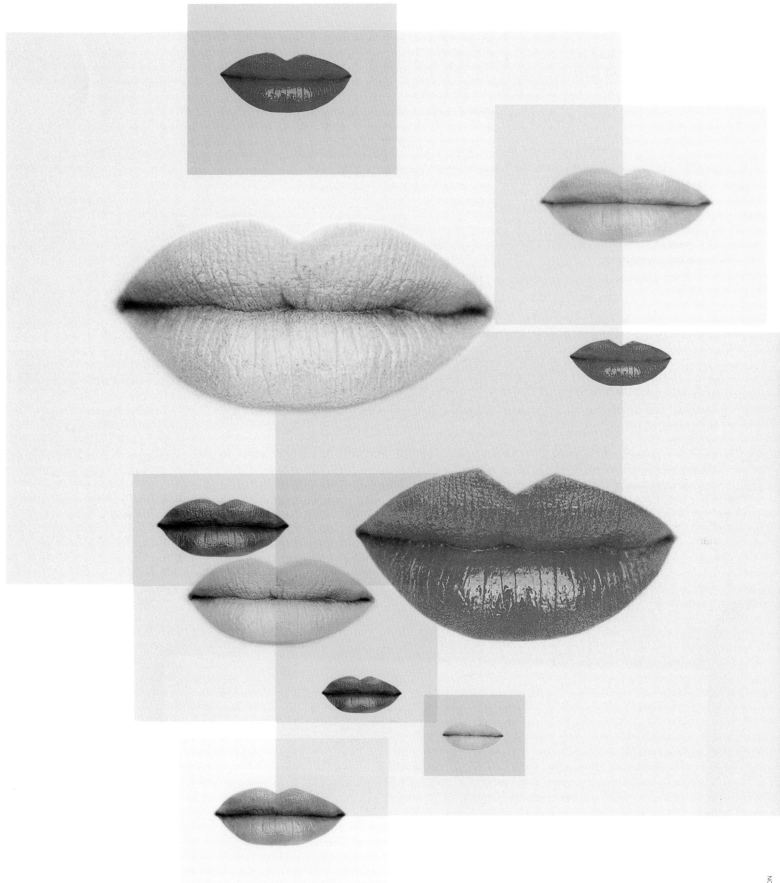

- Some people like the control that a lip brush gives them, but I find it takes too much time. I will carefully line my lips, but then slick on lipstick straight from the tube.
- Lip pencil can double as an ultralong-lasting base for lip color, with a light dab of gloss.
- Gloss is really flattering for older lips because it creates a "soft focus" effect and the illusion of fuller lips. Lancôme has a great gloss called Lip Brio; I also love Make Up For Ever's gloss #6, in a fudgey brown shade (see Resources).
- A dab of gloss in the center of the top and bottom lips creates a fuller look. (Try a hint of silver or gold for evening.) Be careful never to extend gloss beyond the edge of your lipline onto the skin, though; that doesn't look like bigger lips—it looks like sweaty skin.
- In the summer or in warmer climates, the lighter, brighter colors in the pink-peach-coral range are more flattering and help light up your face. Watch what different colors do for your skin tone. I can't wear a blue-red or mauvey red, but orangey reds are perfect for me. If a color makes you look sallow or pale or too pink-skinned, try switching to another shade.
- A skim of shimmer over lips—or over your lipstick—can be very pretty, especially with a suntan (a fake one, of course!). The new shimmery shades are a quantum cosmetics leap from the heavy '60s frosts: they give a veil of color and are great for updating an existing lipstick. Try just a touch of silver, gold, or copper over your favorite color for a wonderful change. A new lipstick is the fastest way to update your look.
- During the day, always carry the color you are wearing for touch-ups, because lipstick is easily disturbed, especially by eating and drinking. If you're wearing a red lipstick, you might want to opt for a stay-put formulation—L'Oréal has a great one called Colour Endure, which even lasts through mealtimes.

TIP

It's very aging and distracting when a woman has lipstick smears on her teeth, but this is a problem which is easily avoided. The classic way is to blot your lipstick with a Kleenex, biting down onto it so that the excess color comes off on the tissue. Another way that's virtually foolproof is to put your forefinger into your mouth, close your lips gently around it, and pull outwards. This action will take off the excess lipstick that's closest to the teeth, without disturbing the rest of your lipcolor.

GETTING THE
BALANCE RIGHT

The tendency, as we get older, is to pile on more makeup. In fact, the older you get, the less you should wear; there's nothing more aging on an older woman than caked-on makeup. Don't play up all of your features at once. If you want to go heavier on the eyes, lighten up the lips—or vice versa. I tend to put blush on right at the end, because you can tell exactly how much you need to balance the rest of your face and finish your look.

The trick with makeup is to look like you're not wearing any. It's important to wear the appropriate makeup for the time of day or the event, but most of all, your makeup must enhance and flatter you. Also, it's crucial not to get stuck over time in exactly the same look. You should make little adjustments every season—a new eyeshadow, a different texture of lipstick; it keeps you up to date and stops you from getting stuck in a time warp!

• Always check your makeup in daylight. (That's also the best place to apply it, if possible.) What your bathroom mirror says is not the truth, because the lighting in bathrooms tends to distort colors or overlight the face.
• Most importantly, make sure all the edges where your makeup ends (shadow, blush and even foundation) are smooth. It sometimes helps to take a cotton ball or pad and lightly buff the face to soften the finished makeup—it blends everything in: around the hairline, under the chin, along the jaw.
• Alternatively, whisk just the tiniest, tiniest touch of blush all over the face, to blur the lines and balance the look.

It's never too late to learn new tricks or perfect your makeup skills. Makeup isn't surgery; it washes right off. It's fun to play and experiment with new techniques, new colors, new tricks—and you should never stop enjoying the fun of it.

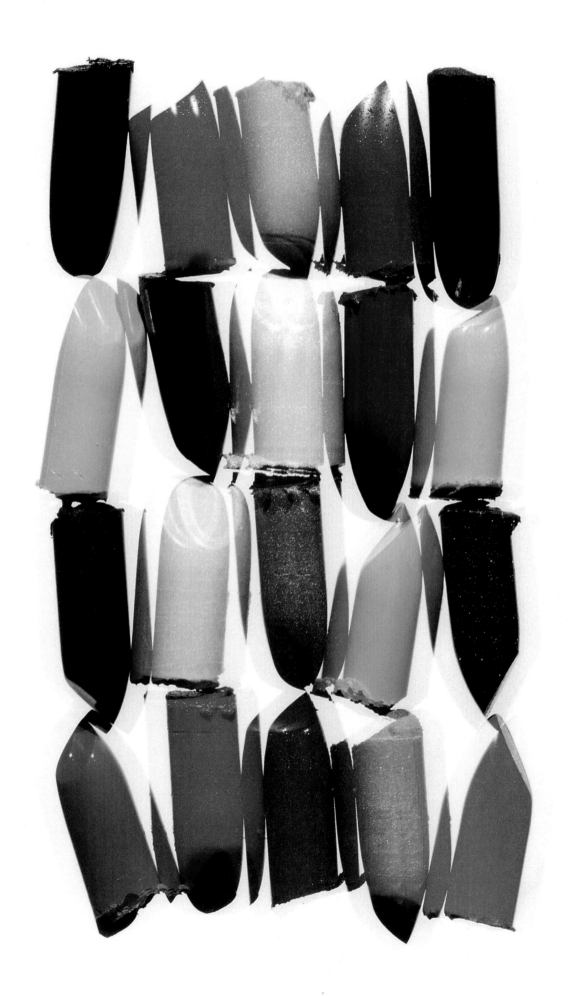

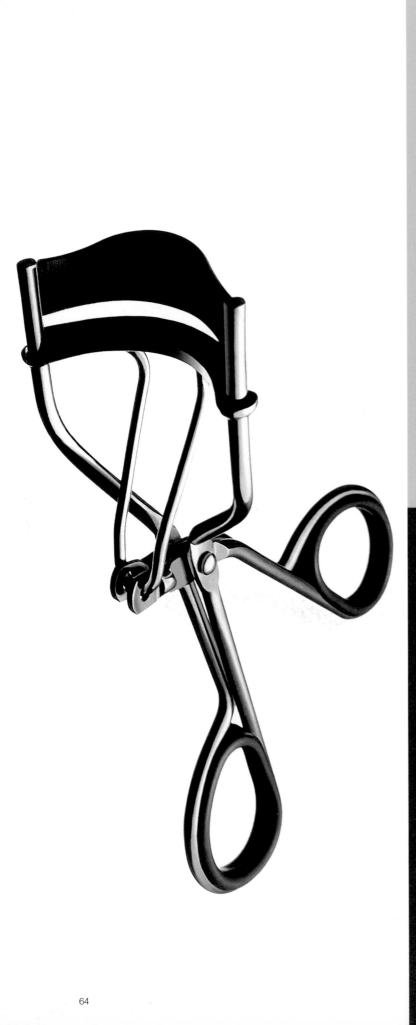

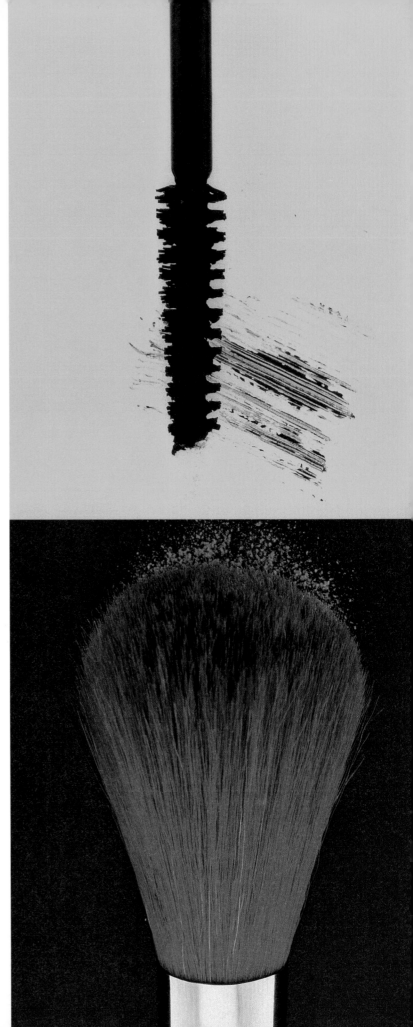

THE ULTIMATE TOOLKIT

What you want is the minimum that does the maximum. I certainly don't like to be encumbered by a lot of makeup. I don't want to lug it around or be confused by it. Best of all, I like makeup that has a double duty. So here's what I've found after years in the business. These are the essentials!

A BLUSH BRUSH Not too short, not so long that it doesn't fit into your makeup bag. It should be fairly flat, rather than round and full, and not too large, because you want to be able to control where the blush is going. If you press the edge of the brush down on a flat surface, the bristles should fan in a half-circle. Always test brushes on the top of your hand; they should feel really, really soft. I've discovered a wonderful range of brushes by Ilise Harris; she uses synthetic hair instead of animal hair. I can usually tell when other makeup artists use her brushes on my skin because they are so soft. But Ilise's brushes are also longer lasting and more hygienic because the synthetic hairs aren't hollow.

A FLAT, FLUFFY BRUSH If you like to use loose powder, you'll need a brush that is even bigger than your blush brush. (If you prefer the pressed variety, it usually comes with a sponge puff or a velvet puff.)

EYE SHADING BRUSHES:

A SMALL POWDER BRUSH Straight-ended or slanted, for eye shading. I use a MAC 22, just to fill in the gaps in my brow with powder shadow.
A TINY, POINTED BRUSH for lining your eyes (my favorite is Laura Mercier No. 2). You need to test it wet and dry, at the counter, if you can: Wet powder shadow makes a more definite line, but some brushes don't pick up shadow well when wet.
A SLIGHTLY FATTER EYESHADOW BRUSH I like Shu Uemura No. 10, for blending powder shadow on my lid.

TWEEZERMAN SLANT TWEEZERS The brand all the makeup artists use.

MAKEUP Foundation (sample bottle for touch-ups), mascara, brown shadow, blush, powder, favorite lipstick or gloss

MIRROR, MIRROR Once over forty, you can't live without a magnifying mirror; it's at the top of my must-have list, an essential for the baby boomer with failing eyesight! I get mine at Zitomer's Pharmacy, in New York (see Resources); department stores also have a great selection. They really do help you see what you're doing. Once you get over the initial shock of seeing everything magnified, you can spot what you've missed, where you overdid it, how to blend, or where the powder got caught in a wrinkle. I gave magnifying mirrors to all my girlfriends one Christmas and they tell me they can't live without them!

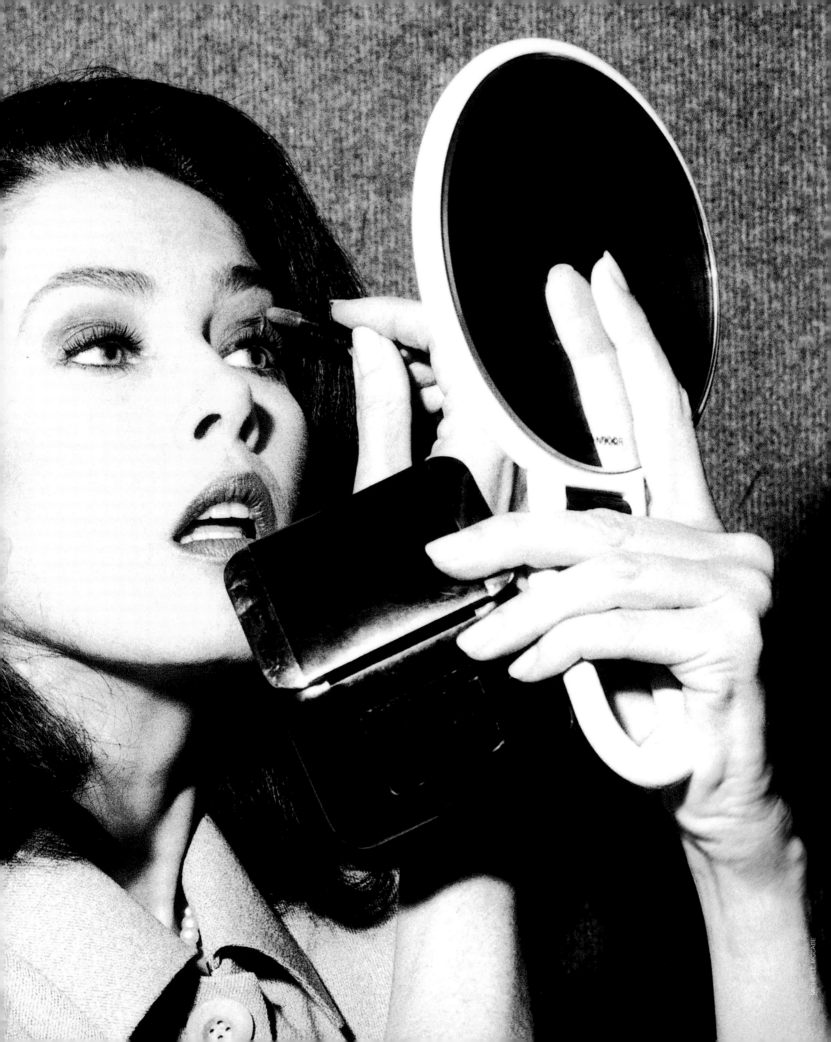

DAY INTO NIGHT MAKEUP

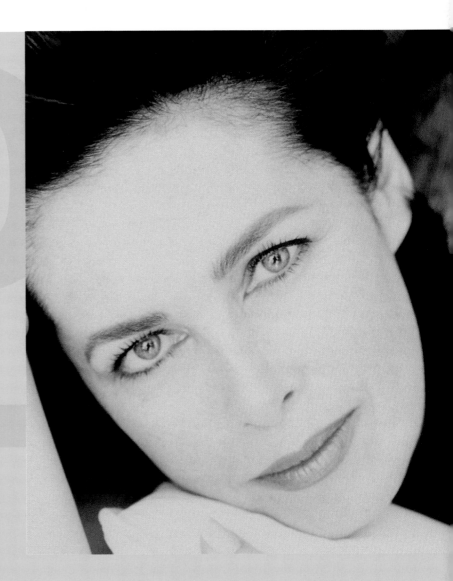

THE TWO MINUTE FACE

Your fast, "emergency" fix when you can't face-the-world-without-at-least-a-little-makeup...

1   Always apply makeup with clean fingers to a moisturized face.
2   Take a tiny dab of your foundation and put a touch under one eye, then the other, on either side of the nose, and underneath the corners of the mouth—so there are six dots altogether.
3   Blend the base lightly with your fingers where you need a little extra coverage—perhaps over broken veins or on under-eye shadows. Don't attempt to cover the whole face.
4   Whisk translucent loose powder lightly over the entire face to even skin tone, yet leave a natural, translucent glow.
5   Using a flat, round brush, whoosh blush over your cheekbones. Remember: think circles, not stripes—and keep the blush high on your cheekbone, almost up to your temples.
6   Slick on a lipstick.
7   Feather the upper lashes with mascara.
8   If you have dark brows, use the last trace of mascara that's on the wand to color them.

DON'T FORGET to moisturize your neck. You can have beautiful makeup but if your neck is dry, it ruins the effect.

DON'T bother with eyeliner; it takes too long. (But if you do want a quickie liner with good control, try L'Oréal Super Liner, which is as easy to use as a felt tip pen).

DO keep all the elements of your two-minute face in a pretty cup in your bathroom, so you can grab for them in a hurry; 1-2-3 . . . Go!

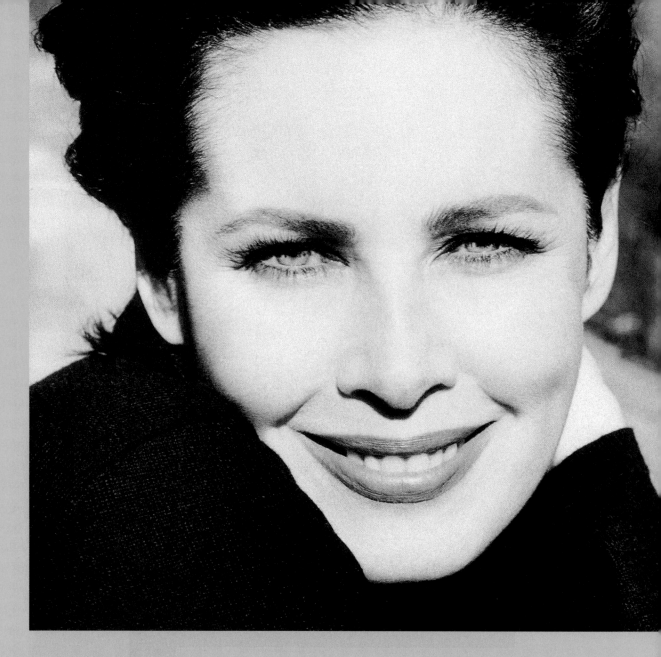

THE FIVE-MINUTE FACE

For your everyday great look. Follow the same steps as in the two-minute face—and build on it by finishing up with these steps:

1   Line your eyes with a dark powder shadow, top and bottom. (Remember: wetting the powder makes the liner last longer).
2   Use the same brush to fill in your brows (always thinking "up").
3   Outline your lips with a lip pencil, then lightly blur the line with your finger.
4   Apply lipstick or lip gloss.

THE TEN-MINUTE FACE

All it takes to glow beautifully in the evening . . .
Follow the instructions for the five-minute face, but take a touch more care and time with every step. Even a great evening look shouldn't take you much more than ten minutes, but techniques are slightly different for serious after-dark occasions. You want an extra-special look, but you don't want thick makeup, so spend a little extra time layering it on subtly.

1   Use a bit more foundation to cover the face, taking the base out to the edge of your face; blend it very carefully into the jawline so there are no visible edges.
2   Make your eye line a little darker—and more precise.

3   Spend a little extra time grooming and filling in your brows.
4   Apply mascara to both your top and bottom lashes, with extra layers at the outer edges.
5   For really grand evenings—a winter ball, a summer soiree—put shimmer on your shoulders, your breastbone, even on your back, wherever your skin is revealed. You can also add a touch of shimmer to your brow bone or on your cheekbone (steering clear of any fine laugh lines).
6   For a nighttime look, use a different eyeshadow on your lids, perhaps a dark mauve-burgundy shade or a sexy smooth gray for extra sultriness.
7   False lashes don't have to make you look like Tammy Faye Baker. The effect of a couple of individual lashes—you can buy them in a strip, or as singles—really opens the eyes. Start from the middle or the outer edge and avoid applying any lashes to the inner half of the eye; you want to emphasize the outer corner, for an eye-opening effect. It's helpful to alternate between eyes, so that the results are perfectly balanced. Space the lashes out; don't clump them together.

DON'T overdo it. Too much makeup is extremely aging. If you are wearing a red lipstick, don't overemphasize your eyes. If you play up your eyes, opt for a slightly subtler lip color. The rule is: *either* dramatic eyes *or* dramatic lips. Never both.

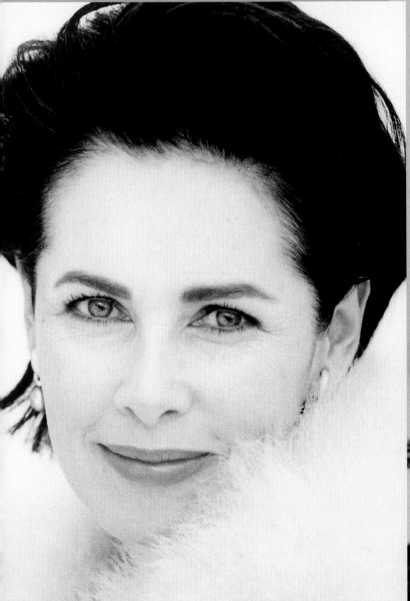

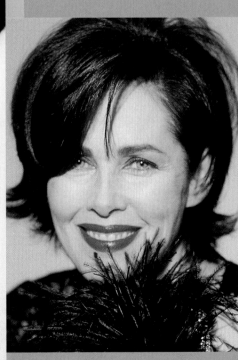

CONFIDENCE-BOOSTING HAIR

3

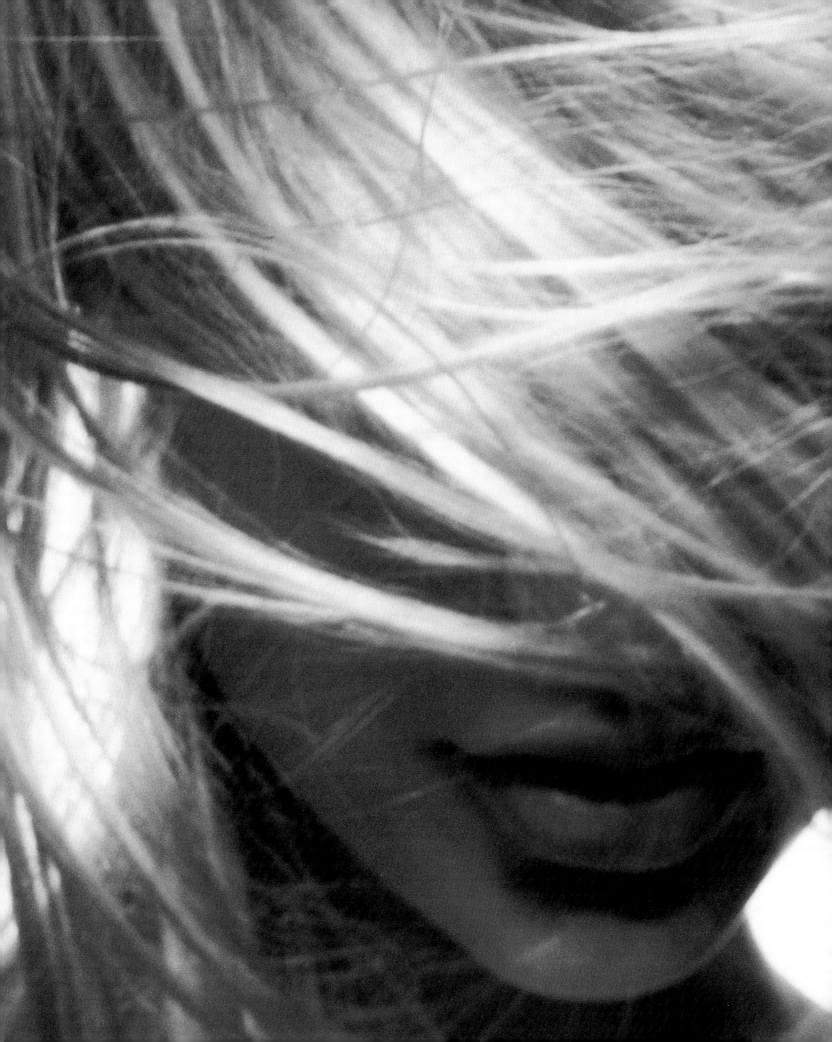

AGE APPROPRIATE HAIR

Great hair is a make-it-or-break factor when it comes to confidence. If our hair is limp and lackluster, fuzzy or frizzy, if we end up with a bad haircut or color job, it can dramatically affect our mood. (The famous bad hair day or week or month!) Both women and men are ultrasensitive about their hair, at every age. Angry or blue—it can show in our hair.

Great-looking hair doesn't have to be time-consuming. What's most important, as we hit our forties and fifties, is to have *age-appropriate* hair. By now we've all experimented. Tried every color under the sun. Been long, been short. But midage is about finding a cut and color that fits and enhances our lifestyle—with the minimum amount of upkeep, because we have better things to do with our time.

Personally, I've found that shorter hair works best for me now. I made one last, die-hard attempt to have long hair recently—but I'm thoroughly enjoying my shorter look. Since I went shorter, my life is so much easier. I spend infinitely less time on hair maintenance. The look appears effortless . . . and it really is! (I'm tired of those "natural" looks that take three hours to achieve!) In a pinch, I can go three or four months between haircuts—yet the style still looks great.

More and more women are going shorter and looking fabulous. Think about how stunning Candice Bergen and Diane Sawyer looked when they cut their hair. Or remember the great change in Barbara Walters when she modernized her look, trading in "pouffy" for sleek. Or Katie Couric, who decided to go really short, creating an innovative look for television. Or Isabella Rossellini and Sharon Stone, who put the focus on their gorgeous faces with minimalist hair. So have fun. Experiment and take risks. If you've had long hair and feel it's time to go shorter, but are afraid of the shock, have it cut in stages—so your eye and self-image can adjust to the new lengths. You might find, as I did, that shorter hair is easier, more flattering, and more fabulous than you ever imagined!

There are exceptions to the as-you-get-older short hair rule, of course. My sister Darilyn is very exotic-looking and has always worn her long hair down or in a braid—and it really suits her. Long hair also saves her a lot of time because all she has to do is tie it back and it changes her look. Think of Georgia O'Keeffe, who made a stunning gray braid into a style signature. Jade Hobson, the fashion editor of New York magazine, has the most beautiful long white hair; it has become her trademark. For many Native American women and women from India, long hair is part of their cultural heritage, and it looks beautiful. These are exceptions that work, creating a strong personal look. A classic trademark style kept over the years can work for certain women who are very sure of themselves: Think of Jackie O., who basically had the same hairstyle for thirty years or more

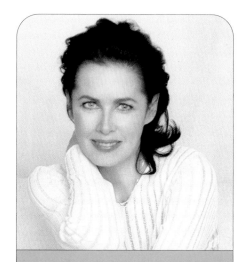

IT'S ABOUT TIME . . .

. . . to make bad hair days a thing of the past. Fortysomething brings new hair challenges: shifts in color and texture. We can live with them, learn to love them—or take advantage of technology to reverse them. Working with some of the world's greatest hair stylists and colorists—and being blessed with hard-to-manage hair— I've watched and observed while they've worked pure magic with cut, colors, styling. Let me share that experience with you now.

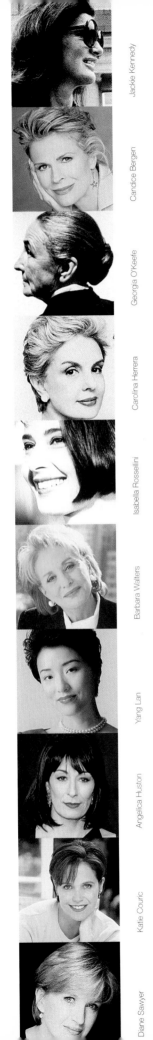

Jackie Kennedy

Candice Bergen

Georgia O'Keefe

Carolina Herrera

Isabella Rossellini

Barbara Walters

Yang Lan

Angelica Huston

Katie Couric

Diane Sawyer

without ever looking old-fashioned or dated. This is not a case of waking up at fifty and suddenly declaring: "A long braid would be nice."

There are some looks that are truly unflattering. One is a tight-curled permanent, which makes everyone look older than they are. If you need extra body, there are body permanents available now that don't result in that poodle-curl look. The wrong hair color can also add years; color that's too orangey brown and brassy, or coal black hair if it's not your natural color (see You Don't Have to Go Gray, Even Gracefully, Page 82, for how to avoid these mistakes).

One of the secrets to finding a great hairstyle, though, is to talk, talk, talk to your hairdresser before he flashes his scissors (let alone any chemicals). Hairdressers should always offer a free, no-commitment consultation before you book an appointment for a cut. Communicate to your hairdresser your lifestyle: how much time you have for upkeep—and describe your personal style. (It may help for them to see you in your street clothes first, rather than an anonymous salon gown.) Do you really want a cut that needs to be blown dry every few days?

I believe that paying for a great haircut can be a better investment than buying a new dress, because your hair frames your face and is something you wear *every* day. Sometimes, it takes a trip to a different hairdresser to get a new look that works for you. Your own tried-and-trusted hairdresser may see you only in a certain way. Tear out cuts and styles you like from magazines and take them along when you talk with your hairstylist. (If he's offended, change stylists.)

One fact you may not know is that hair texture changes as we age. Gray hair tends to be coarser and wirier than hair with natural color. Perming and coloring hair also alters the texture; these processes affect the hair shaft, plumping up the individual hairs. This thickening of the hair is actually a bonus because as we get older, most of us tend to experience thinning hair. If your hair is developing more gray or if you've just begun to have it colored, then this is a good time to rethink your style, to make the most out of these shifts in texture.

If I have a problem, I will always ask my hairdresser for hints. "How do you do that?" Or "What's the best new product for this or that?" One trick that hairdressers can teach every one of us is how to use Velcro rollers. They're such a blessing—and a quantum advance from the old-fashioned wire ones with clips. They're amazingly useful if you have thin hair because they help create instant volume.

RESCUE REMEDY   A few years ago I experienced a hair disaster beyond belief. I had my hair straightened—and ended up with a fried, broken, dead mop. It was a bad dream come true. A nightmare. In a panic (and after an emergency trim), I went to see Philip B., who's a hair-repair miracle worker. He prescribed his Philip B. Botanical Oil (see Resources), and with just a single treatment, he restored a lot of the gloss and helped my hair come back to life. Nowadays, if my hair feels or looks dry, I just rub a couple of drops of his special oil into my hands and scrunch it into the ends of my hair. It gives my hair great texture, definition, and shine—instantly. Alternatively, if your ends are beyond redemption, you'll need to have them trimmed off and keep trimming until your

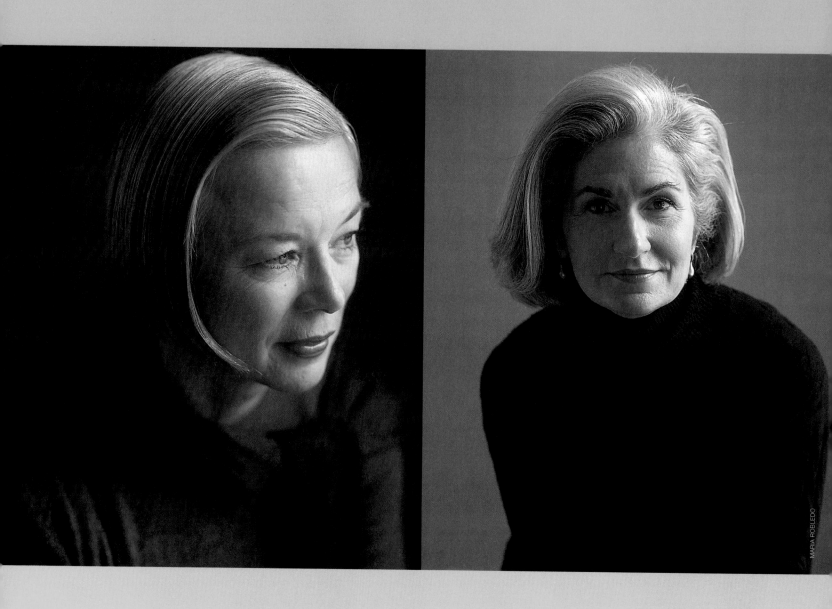

hair looks and feels healthy and terrific. Be conscious that all chemical treatments affect your hair's condition. You'll need to put back in what the chemicals take out. Remember: shiny hair is young-looking hair.

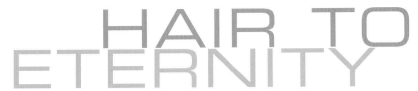

HAIR TO ETERNITY

All of you blessed straight-haired readers . . . BYPASS THIS SECTION. This is not for you. This chapter is for those of us who must face the challenge of curly and frizzy hair on a day-to-day basis. We all know who we are!

As a teenager, I remember staring enviously at photographs of girls in the magazines with long blonde hair, like sheets down their bodies, defying the forces of nature. This was the '60s. They had bangs and length. I had curls that never grew. I tried taping my bangs to my forehead, ironing my stubborn curls, and sleeping in soup can rollers—all in an attempt to achieve the lovely, silky lengths that effortlessly mocked me from the glossy pages.

It is not easy laying your head on an ironing board, stretching your hair to its full, glorious two-inch length with one hand and trying to iron it with the other. But iron I did, often burning my hair, my fingers, and, occasionally, a very unhappy ear. Neither of my sisters had this hair affliction and they watched me with great amusement and an even greater pity.

Eventually, I developed a method of wrapping my hair completely around my head and rolling the top of it with two full-size soup cans, enveloping the whole thing in a lovely blue hairnet. It was a delightful sight and not one I allowed many people to see.

CURLY HAIR MASTER CLASS To keep curly hair like mine perfectly under control, here are my secrets:

1   When hair is wet, put a dab of hair gel—about the size of a dime—in the palm of the hand (for medium-length hair, a nickel-sized dab; for long hair, a quarter-sized dab).
2   With two fingers, take a touch of gel and gently pat it around the hairline, where hair tends to get the frizziest frizzes.
3   Rub the rest of the gel in your hands, spreading it all through your hair—paying special attention to the ends.
4   Lightly spritz hair relaxer all over the hair to relax and smooth the curl. (I have a special one from Stephen Knoll in New York that I just love—see Resources.)
5   Blow out hair on the outside of a round brush, pulling firmly from the root to the ends, section by section.
6   Style from the top of your head working to the bottom, putting each dry section of hair in a hair velcro roller to hold its shape and get it out of the way.

7 Starting from the top again, unwind each roller, taking a hot electric flat iron and ironing each section. Then re-roll the section, to take out any left over frizz. (This takes a bit of maneuvering, but once you're adept at it, the process takes less than five minutes.)

8 After you've removed the rollers, take a dime-sized dollop of hair cream. Rub it between the hands and lightly, lightly feather the fingers along the top hairs of the entire head. With the bit that is left on the fingers, gently pull the ends of your hair. This gives weight to the hair and stops it from fluffing up on humid days. This is also an opportunity to shape your hair finally with the cream.

9 To leave nothing to frizz-fate, as you dress, pin the two sides close to your head with long-handled silver clips to sleek it in place; as the heat goes out of the hair, it sets, keeping the head "small."

DAY TO DAY
HAIRCARE

In the quest for great hair, it's possible to squander a fortune on hair-styling gizmos and products. Over the years, though, I've had the chance to try most of what is out there—and here's what I can't live without:

- VELCRO ROLLERS Blue, red, and pink (different sizes for different lengths of hair). Right now, while my hair's really short, I tend to use the blue rollers most often. I travel with the Velcro curlers, packed one inside the other; if my hair gets flattened by sleeping, I pop in a couple of rollers in the morning, jump in the shower, and let the steam set my hair. Voilá—instant body and bounce!

- LONG-HANDLED SILVER HAIR CLIPS These are useful for keeping hair off the face when applying makeup. I also like to use them to clip the sides of my hair for a sleeker effect if it has too much body after blow drying—sometimes spritzing as well, to flatten the hair. (That overly "round," blow-dried look tends to be old-fashioned.) I'll keep the clips in until I have to go out.

- A HOT FLAT IRON A must for transforming curly, frizz-prone hair into a smoother look. Babyliss makes irons that come in several sizes, including one that's portable, for traveling. (Again, ask your hairdresser to show you how to use one; you don't want to overdo it and damage your hair.)

- MURRAY'S WAX This is a product for grooming Afro-American hair that you can find at any drugstore. Just a tiny, tiny dab on the end of your fingers is all you need—otherwise hair gets too greasy. Run a tiny bit lightly along the top of your hair to smooth strays and add weight; or run the wax through your hair to "break hair up"—giving it texture and control without oiliness. You can also apply a bit of Murray's to the ends to shape your hair.

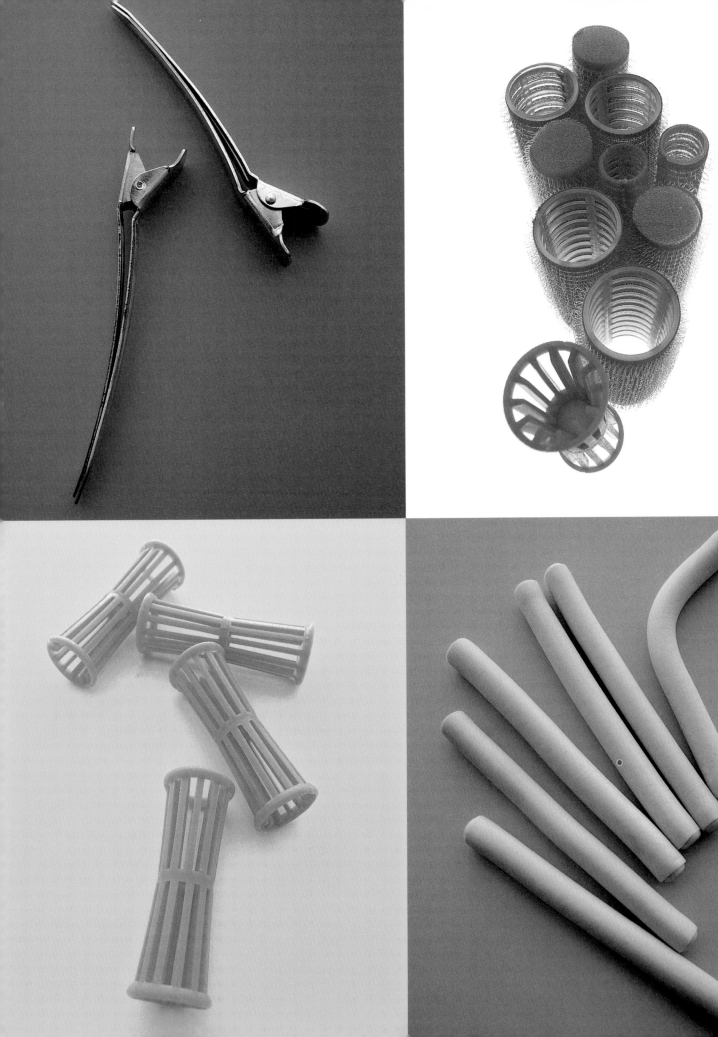

- PHYTODEFRISANT STRAIGHTENING BALM Before you style your hair, apply a dollop into your wet hair and comb through (with a wide-tooth comb) to make sure it's evenly distributed. This straightening balm penetrates the hair shaft and smoothes out the curls, catching the frizz before it begins. I love it (see Resources)!

- STEPHEN KNOLL'S TOTALLY AMAZING TRANSFORMING SPRAY This spray can be used on curly, frizzy, or coarse hair. You need just a tiny amount; it helps straighten out hair and controls it—literally transforming rather than giving stiff hold.

- KIEHL'S SILK GROOM Just the tiniest dot, rubbed into the palms of the hands and skimmed over the hair, controls flyaway hair and gives the perfect weight to my hair. If you've got really, really fine hair, be careful—it can make it too greasy (see Resources).

- CONAIR HAIRDRYERS Mine is a great, sturdy 1600-watt version. (Hairdressers always use 1600 or above.) You must be certain to secure the little nozzle attachment that directs the flow, otherwise you can burn hair and even damage the scalp.

- L'ORÉAL VIVE SHAMPOOS AND CONDITIONERS These products give hair fabulous shine and body. Frédéric Fekkai's line is terrific too; he has a deliciously scented lemon rinse that's very light, yet conditioning (see Resources). I also love Philip B.'s Peppermint Shampoo, which makes the scalp tingle—a great morning wake-up!

- A TERRY CLOTH–LINED SHOWER CAP This is another must—it keeps out the humidity on the days you shower without shampooing. Steam from the shower is the "hair enemy": It makes curly hair frizz and causes straight hair to flatten. I'd be a perpetual poodle without my cap.

- DIFFERENT SIZES OF ROUND BRISTLE BRUSHES Great for styling hair. (Your hairdresser may be the best source for professional-quality styling brushes.) I also like a wide-toothed comb for combing hair while it's wet. You should never tug wet hair because it can split and break. Think of wet hair as being as fragile as old lace—and treat it gently. (A very thin, inexpensive comb with a metal tail is also useful because you can use the tail of the comb to separate hair, to put rollers in or to apply color.)

HAIR IN THE SUN

Exposure to sunshine is a disaster for hair—especially older hair, which is drier, less resilient, and probably chemically treated. (If colored brunette hair is exposed to the sun, it develops a reddish tinge almost instantly.) So I have an armory of hair protectants. I wear a wide-brimmed hat on sunny days—and a silk headscarf even when the day isn't so bright. (The silk has a polishing effect on hair, too.) There are also terrific hair protectors to pack for vacations: J. F. Lazartigue and Phytomer both make sunscreens for hair that help protect against the damaging effects of chlorine. They're both quite oily-textured, so if you don't want to slick your hair down, simply rub the regular body sunscreen in the palms of your hands and skim it over the top of your hair.

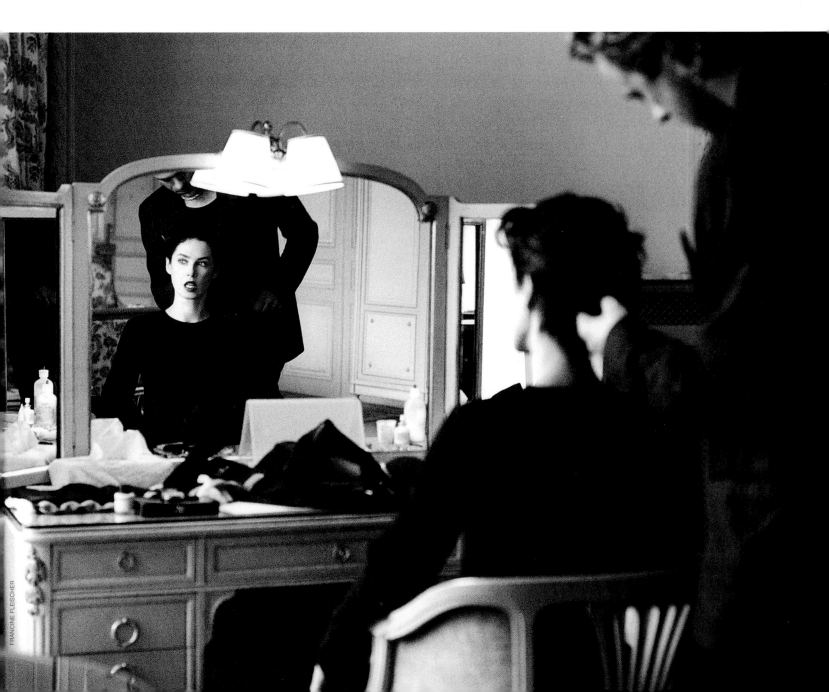

FRANCINE FLEISCHER

THE RIGHT INGREDIENTS FOR YOUR
HAIR TYPE

Some ingredients in shampoos, conditioners, and styling products are better for different hair types than others. Use the wrong ones and your hair may get flat quicker, look lank, or simply not get the moisture it needs to combat frizz. Just as you probably look at the ingredients on food labels, start to scan the ingredients list of shampoos, conditioners, and styling products to make sure you're getting the right match for your hair type.

FINE TO NORMAL

You want products that won't weigh down hair and make it look flatter than it usually is; fine hair can appear flat easily.

You want to use shampoos with:
polyquaterniums
hydrolyzed proteins
copolymers

Look for rinse-out conditioners featuring:
carbomers
proteins
amino acids

In styling aids, seek out products that feature:
water
alcohol
resins
copolymers
and the words
firm, *high*, or *maximum hold*,
but use sparingly

NORMAL TO COARSE

What you're after are products that will add shine and help you control hair.

Try to use products that contain:
lanolins
oils
words ending in *methicone*,
plus hydrolyzed proteins

Rinse-out conditioners should contain:
anthenol
oils
cholesterol
shea butter
ingredients ending in *one*

When it comes to styling products, look for those with built-in conditioning and shine-boosting ingredients.
The key ingredients are:
silicone
oils
resins
plant mucilage
the words *gentle* or *moisturizing*

HAIR PRODUCTS DEMYSTEFIED

There's an arsenal of hair-care products out there — and for those of us who grew up when just about all there was to keep our hair in place was Dippity-Do, the choices can be baffling. So here's the low-down on what does what, to help steer you towards the best products for your hair — and style.

DE-FRIZZERS are useful for curly hair, preventing a flyaway look by relaxing and controlling hair. They often come in the form of a silicone-based serum, which coats the hair and should be used sparingly on wet hair only. Infusium 23 is a great leave-in spray that can be found in any drugstore.

GELS are useful for giving body to fine to medium hair, but must be used very sparingly. (Often, a nickel-sized squirt of gel is all you need.) They are best when applied to washed hair, when your hair is 70 to 80 percent dry.

MOUSSES are good for giving volume, although in my experience some mousses can dull hair. Look for those that are alcohol-free and contain vitamins or other conditioning ingredients. Mousses give hold and volume to hair. Like gels, they are best applied to hair that's 70 to 80 percent dry.

SPRAYS are useful for holding hair in place, but do be careful to pick a product that gives natural-looking results—and never overdo it! Hair that looks like it's been "fixed" is old-fashioned and aging. Also, look for those products that help to condition or give gloss to hair as well as hold it. Some of the sprays I like are L'Oréal Elnett (it's been around for years in Europe; I love the old-fashioned smell . . . and it works!) and Stephen Knoll's Perfect Holding Mist. These sprays let your hair move and add a little conditioning shine, while holding the look you want in place.

TEXTURIZING LOTIONS give a wonderful tousled effect that makes hair look more modern and young. (Think of Meg Ryan's hair: That's great texture.) Put a dab in your hands, rub them together, and scrunch the ends of your hair. A word of caution: Add the product slowly to gauge how your hair adapts to it. Texturizing lotions are usually for hair that's 70 to 80 percent dry.

VOLUMIZERS do what they say—so they're great for hair that tends to go flat. They can be applied to wet hair or to hair that's partially dry, depending on the formulation. As women age, a little extra volume can be more flattering and give extra oomph to thinning hair, so that you don't see the scalp.

WAXES are great for giving texture, "breaking up" hair that's been blow-dried, to give it more definition. They enable you to sculpt your hair. A tiny dot of wax, rubbed between the palms, can be sleeked over hair, or used on the ends of individual curls. Experiment.

POMADES are lighter than waxes and wash out more easily, so they give similar results but are more manageable. A pomade, like a wax, needs a little practice—just a little goes a long way. You can see the effects of pomades or wax in photos of many actresses, like Demi Moore, Winona Ryder, and Courteney Cox. For a woman in her forties, a pomade can be a helpful tool to smooth frizz at the ends of the hair, to control a "too-bouffant" look (which is aging), or to weigh and sculpt the ends of the hair in the direction you wish them to go (e.g., bangs or even split ends).

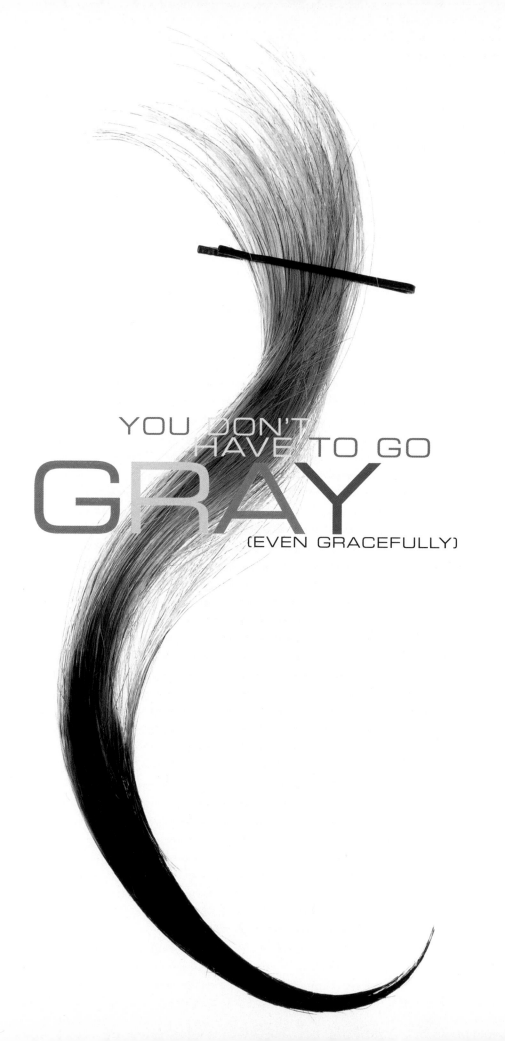

YOU DON'T
HAVE TO GO
GRAY
(EVEN GRACEFULLY)

ILAN RUBIN

Coloring my hair was something I resisted for many years. At the time, I thought that coloring my hair was cheating. That is, until the day I was being photographed for Harper's Bazaar in Rome, wearing fabulous Valentino gowns, and the hairdresser couldn't quite cover what nature was boldly revealing—my gray! I quickly came to the realization that coloring my hair would be exciting; it would simply mean I was taking care of myself.

Some people however, go gray beautifully. There are several models in the fashion business, such as stunning sixtysomething Carmen Del'Orefice and prematurely gray Marie Seznac (designer Christian Lacroix muse), and Harper's Bazaar Editor-in-chief LIz Tilberis, whose signature is their stunning steely white hair. In my experience, gray hair can also be striking if your usual style of dress is somewhat ethnic, exotic, or flamboyant. A few women, generally those with pink-cheeked English-rose complexions or deep ebony skin, look head-turningly gorgeous when they go silver; the white hair acts like a photographer's light and highlights the features. But many more women can look sallow, washed out, and just plain older with gray hair. Olive-skinned women rarely find silver hair flattering and natural redheads tend to fade out when white is mixed in.

There's no getting away from it: your first gray hair is a real shocker. And your second and your third. As a result, there are some classic mistakes that women make when it comes to covering up that gray in your forties, fifties, and up. As you age, the tone and texture of your skin changes, so to select the most flattering shade, you should choose a shade slightly lighter than your natural hair color. This will brighten your face, lift your eyes, and enhance your skin tone. I used to have naturally blue-black hair when I was younger and I've had to go lighter and lighter. A too-dark color screams, "Dye job, dye job" and makes you look harsh and older. (I'm sure you've seen men fall into the same trap—with the giveaway jet-black hair that makes them look like Japanese Kabuki dancers.)

As to choosing what type of haircolor you should use, there are several different options:

TEMPORARY COLOR A shampoo-in, shampoo-out color treatment that simply deposits color on the outside of the hair shaft and lasts through a single wash. It can be used to give you temporary coverage and add depth and shine to your hair. Temporary color is most suitable for women with just a few gray hairs. You can use it with permanent color as a color booster, especially red tones, which tend to fade the fastest.

VEGETABLE COLORS While made from crushed and powdered flowers, leaves, fruits, or nuts, the active ingredients are often similar to those found in traditional haircolor. However, I do not recommend them as it is hard to control color consistency, and many of them are drying, especially hennas.

SEMIPERMANENT COLOR This doesn't contain ammonia or peroxide, so these are truly gentle to the hair. Semi-permanents do not lighten hair but can help cover gray, while adding depth and shine to hair. They are also low-commitment because they gradually fade in six to eight shampoos, leaving no visible rootline. Semi-permanent colors are recommended for women with up to 20 percent gray.

Semi-permanent haircolor is a fabulous way of introducing yourself to a particular shade, because it fades naturally in a few shampoos. Loving Care by Clairol was my first hair colorant. I loved it because I could easily shampoo it in, and it disappeared in just six washes. I still use it sometimes, in a pinch, to catch the roots between salon visits.

DEMI-PERMANENT COLOR This lasts approximately six to eight weeks. It contains just a small amount of peroxide to allow the color to penetrate the hair shaft, helping to cover resistent gray and offering a large range of colors. Demi-permanent colors provide better coverage and therefore are suitable for women with up to 50 percent gray. Like semi-permanents, demi-permanents can be used to enhance your color and add shine, or if you use a lighter shade, they can give you a natural highlighted effect.

PERMANENT COLOR This penetrates the hair shaft, giving long-lasting results. It provides great coverage and offers a full range of colors. You can go lighter or darker depending on the shade you choose. However, they can also make hair look flat and monotone, so many top colorists suggest highlighting or lowlighting in addition. It is recommended to touch up your roots and refresh your color every six weeks. However, it is truly dependent on how fast your hair grows and the color contrast between roots and ends. Permanent colors will cover up to 100 percent gray.

HIGHLIGHTS Highlights use bleach (ammonia and peroxide) on selected strands of hair—from fine highlights to funky "chunks"—so the process is permanent. Upkeep is between six weeks to three months, depending on your natural color and rate of new growth.

HELPFUL HAIR HINTS: Here are my tips for haircolor that looks utterly natural, whether coloring hair at home or in a salon:
• Always lighten the section of hair that frames your face a shade or two lighter than the rest of your hair. It helps avoid the harshness of a dyed-hair look and brightens the face, giving it more radiance and youth.
• As you get older, all-over, one-color dark hair simply doesn't look real. It is more effective to break up the color with slightly lighter highlights that are subtle enough to look as if the sun has lifted it naturally. But make sure your hairdresser highlights only tiny strands around the face.
• Take it from someone who's learned from experience: Just seven dollars (the cost of a home hair colorant) and thirty minutes can make you look and feel ten years younger. It's probably the most bang you'll ever get from your buck . . . and your time.

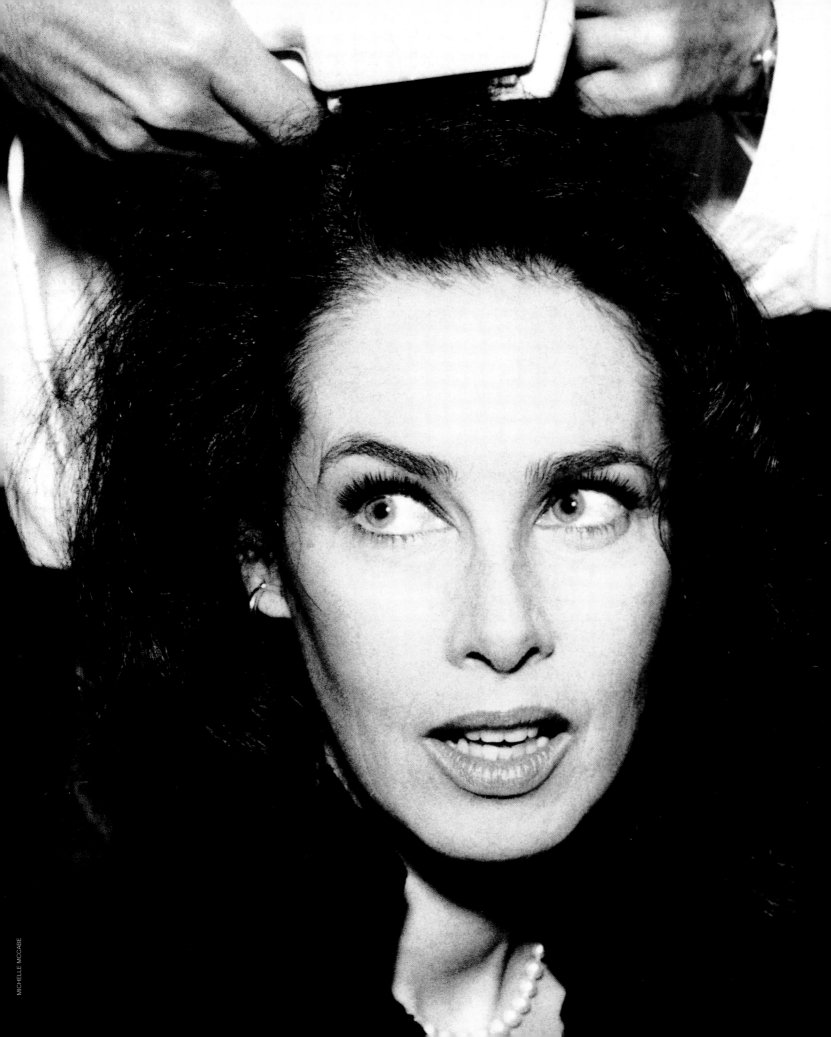

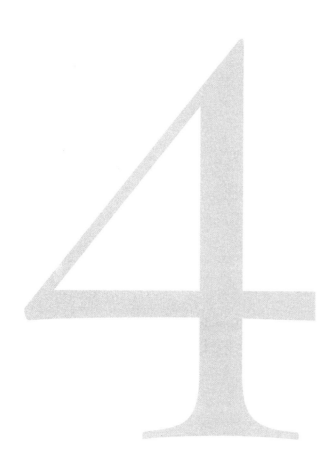

4

BODY TALK

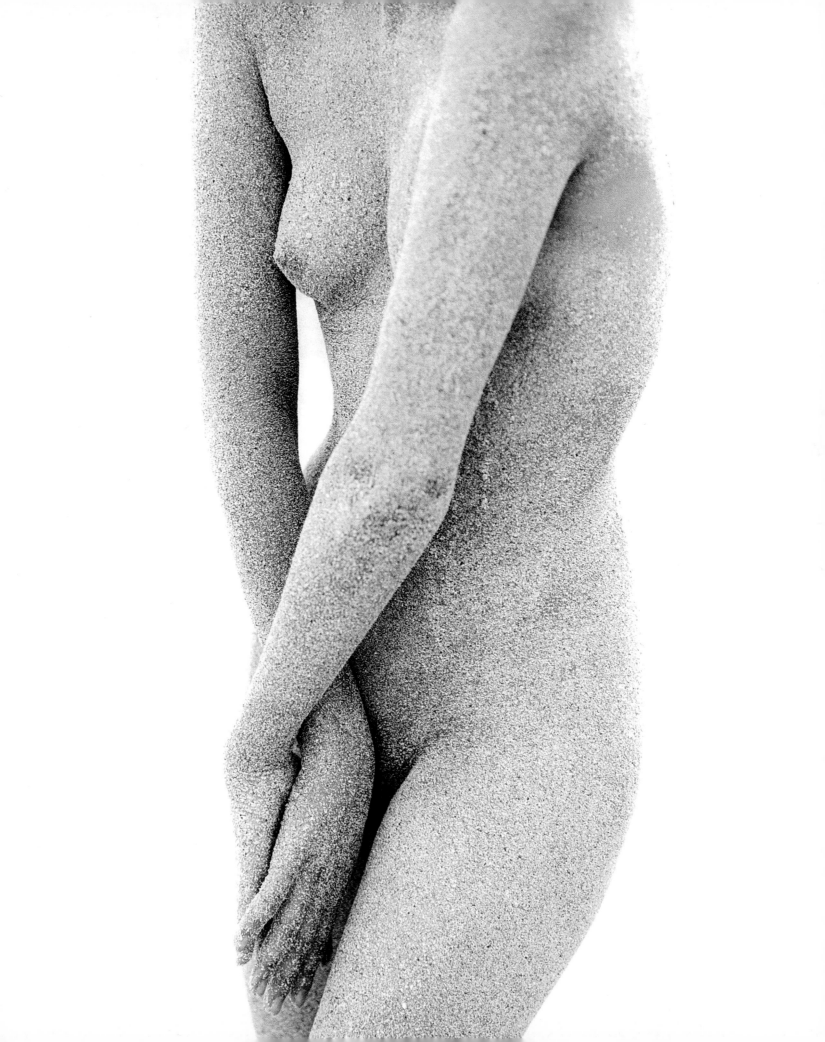

BODYCARE

Our skin, covering us from head to toe, does a perfect job protecting us from the world. It is our body's largest organ and our first line of defense. Amazingly, we also eliminate up to a pound of waste each day through the skin (mostly by perspiring), which is why the skin is sometimes called the "third kidney."

As we hit our forties, our skin has lost some of its elasticity and now needs *extra* care. We can take care of our skin from the inside out by eating in a healthy way, getting enough sleep, and by cultivating a life philosophy that enhances how we feel about ourselves. All of these elements are reflected in how we look. But we can also take care of our bodies from the outside in. What's more, lavishing attention on our bodies helps prevent our skin from looking and feeling dry, dull, and dingy—defying one of aging's unwanted gifts.

BODY BRUSHING   An instant way to give your body and spirit a boost is to dry body brush. The list of body-brushing achievements is extremely impressive. It stimulates the circulation and improves lymphatic flow; the more efficient our lymphatic system, the stronger our immune system. (Many people who practice daily skin brushing actually report fewer ailments like headaches, colds, and flu symptoms.)

Body brushing also helps flush excess water from tissues and so helps combat puffiness and bloating. It makes our skin more supple and increases cell renewal, thus minimizing premature aging of the skin. What's more, I find it gives an instant energy lift and imparts a gorgeous glow. Joyce Ma, a famous figure in the fashion industry, goes so far as to say that body brushing changed her entire body shape—and helped her lose weight.

The best times to brush are morning and before bed. Personally, I like it as an instant wake-up tonic; I find that dry brushing makes me feel as if I've just been for a brisk walk—re-energized, happy, and raring to go.

What equipment do you need? Just a natural body brush. Make sure that the bristles aren't too hard (they will literally scratch skin), or too soft, in which case they'll be ineffective.

If you're not used to body brushing, you might want to start with a medium-soft body brush. Once you're used to brushing, you can move on to a slightly firmer version. You should have your own brush—just as you have your own toothbrush—and wash it every few weeks with soap and water; let it dry naturally in the sun or a dry room. Always brush dry skin, never damp or wet, as this can cause stretching, and avoid any areas that are bruised, irritated, or have wounds.

I start at my toes, working my way up toward the heart. Move upward in quick strokes, starting from the toes and legs, then fingers to shoulders, making sure to always head toward the heart. Body brushes come with long or short handles. With a long-handled brush, it's easier to reach your back. (Or you could ask someone to do it for you!)

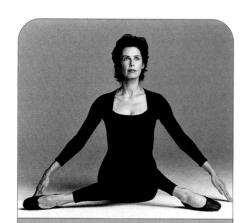

IT'S ABOUT TIME . . .

. . . to realize that a great body is a healthy body. I believe that taking care of our bodies—inside and out— is a must for every woman, a reflection of how good we feel about ourselves. Yes, bodies change over the years. Gravity, calories, and a busy lifestyle take their toll. So at midlife, a great body isn't about aiming for perfection: It's about understanding our bodies, learning to love what we can't fix—and fixing what we can.

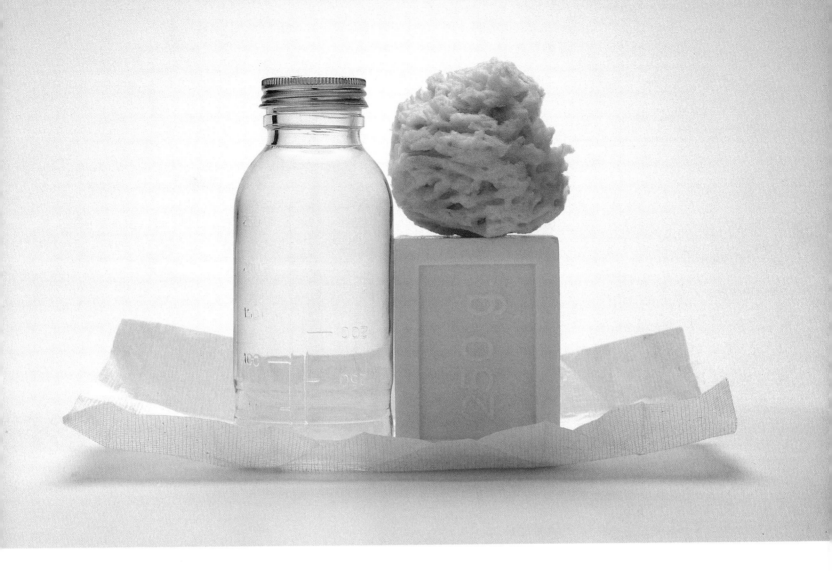

At the end of a particularly stressful day, body brushing can serve as a great relaxer, prepping the body (and the mind) for a great night's sleep. At times, I feel that with body brushing, I can slough off all the wear and tear of the day. Crawling into bed without first taking care of my body feels as if I'm tucking the stress of the entire day in between the covers with me—and that's a little too crowded for my taste!

Head-to-toe exfoliation not only smoothes your skin, it's also very healthy. The skin has an easier time eliminating waste when dead surface cells have been whisked away. I find that if I body brush, my creams and oils can penetrate better, leaving my skin better moisturized and younger looking. I like to keep a very rough cloth by my bath and literally scrub from the tips of my toes and soles of my feet to the neck area, working up and paying special attention to the areas where rough skin tends to build up and get "knobbly": ankles, knees, elbows, and backside (which definitely gets a bum deal from our sedentary lifestyles). Colored nylon mitts are also very effective scrubbers, as are "agave" cloths, which look like they're made of a kind of string, but are in fact woven from a tough, cactus-like plant (available at most specialty bath shops or pharmacies—see Resources).

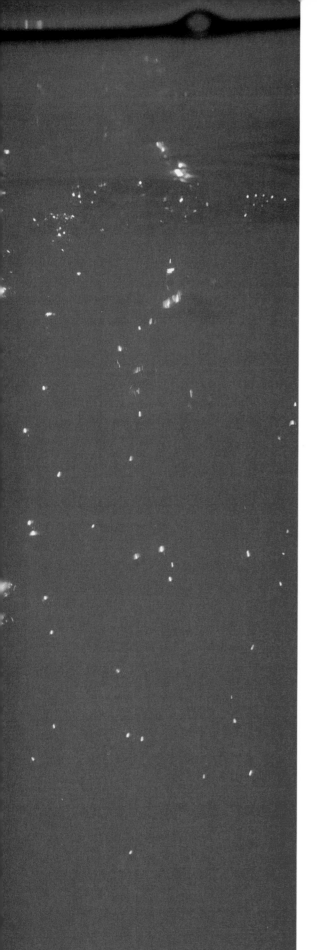

BODY BYTES

- Sometimes I like to briskly rub my entire body with a terry towel while I'm still half wet from a bath or shower. The rubbing back and forth creates a warming friction and basically gets the machine going. You can really feel the wonderful effect this has on your circulation—you'll glow all over!

- I'm a firm believer in the power of touch. I once read that we need nine hugs a day to have a sense of well-being. Well, trust me, I'm working on it! A hug from the right person is totally relaxing and reassuring, creating a feeling of love and acceptance. Massage, of course, has a similar effect; not only does it help melt the body's stresses and tensions away, but it also represents a simple extended human contact—which we all crave. What's more, massage "keeps it all moving."

- As we get older, we can turn back the clock by improving skin quality. Dried-out, uncared-for skin doesn't invite anyone's touch. I'm always experimenting, trying creams, lotions, potions, and oils to lavish onto my skin. Neutrogena makes a wonderful sesame oil that elegantly glides onto and into the skin after a bath; it's light and has a beautiful fragrance. Lancôme's Re-Source is also a fabulous body-care product, an oil that converts into a cream when you spritz it onto the skin. I find health food stores are a great source for body care; almond oil, in particular, is very skin-friendly and moisturizing, without being heavy. Anything that helps improve the skin's barrier function—locking moisture in and preventing evaporation—is great news.

- Skin is mostly water. We are mostly water, and we need to drink a lot of it to keep the body hydrated. Six or seven glasses a day is a great prescription. Dehydration can come on surprisingly quickly, so when you're feeling slow or sluggish, or if you sense a headache coming on, simply drinking a glass of water can yield instant benefits. And skin that's well-moisturized from within looks healthy and glowing on the outside.

- Hands will reveal your age faster than a glance at your driver's license. That's why hands need extra attention—especially in winter, or if you use them a lot. (Women who handle paper tend to have very dry hands—the paper literally absorbs the moisture from the skin. Likewise, women whose hands are often in water must contend with chapped hands.) Neutrogena's Norwegian Formula (mentioned in Problem Spots and Angst Areas, p. 42) provides a great antidote.

- As with the face and neck (see Skin: The Bottom Lines on Lines, p. 22), minimize your body's exposure to the sun at all times. Walk on the shady side of the street and wear wide-brimmed hats that protect your shoulders as well as your face. You may think I'm overzealous on this subject, but believe me, every little bit counts.

- If you must have that bronzed look, then fake it—with a tan in a bottle. Lancôme's range is fantastic: they have a spray-on self-tanner that makes it easier to reach more difficult areas, like your back, and a cream formulation self-tanner which gives a wonderfully even application. Faking it is the best way to control the color and intensity of your tan—and to protect your long-term health and appearance.

- A beautiful pedicure and manicure can distract from other, less-than-perfect parts of the body. My rule is to go wild on the feet—and keep the colors beautifully calm on the hands. Because the hands age so quickly, it isn't always a great idea to draw attention to them. A subtle, quiet look for your nails can be more elegant.

- Longer nails can be a bit aging, although some women have made them a trademark. They tell me that they feel more feminine with longer nails. For nail length, I personally prefer a natural shape, kept fairly short. In our forties and up, we want a natural–colored, simple, clean look to the nails—one that looks great and works with our lifestyle. (But that doesn't mean that we can't break out the red nails when we're in the mood.)

- I will not do my household chores without rubber gloves. Detergents and cleaners are too harsh on the hands and on the nails. Even dusting without gloves dries hands out, so I have little cotton housework gloves. (You can get them from the Vermont Country Store catalog—see Resources, catalog numbers—or look for "cheapo" cotton gloves at a hardware store.) A great hand treatment is to slather a thick layer of cream on your hands, then slide them into cotton gloves, guaranteeing silky-smooth hands by morning. (You can do the same with your feet and a cozy pair of cotton socks.) I also keep gloves in my car, because hands pick up so much sun while driving. Wear gloves in the cold and in the rain. Keep hands out of the elements, at all times, and they'll love you for it. And keep hand cream literally at your fingertips.

- A hand massage is a real tension-buster; we carry a lot of stress in our hands without even realizing it. It's good to bend the hand in both directions, to free up the wrist and give them a good stretch. Wrap one hand around a finger of the opposite hand and pull upward, almost flicking the tension out of the hand. Then massage the hands all over, with a silky, soothing hand cream. (If you really want to indulge, heat up the cream for a couple of seconds in the microwave first.) If you have any leftover cream, rub it into the nail area—which can get very dry, especially in winter—and smooth any remaining cream into your elbows. Hands are often a first impression, so make sure they're smooth, soft, and silky to the touch.

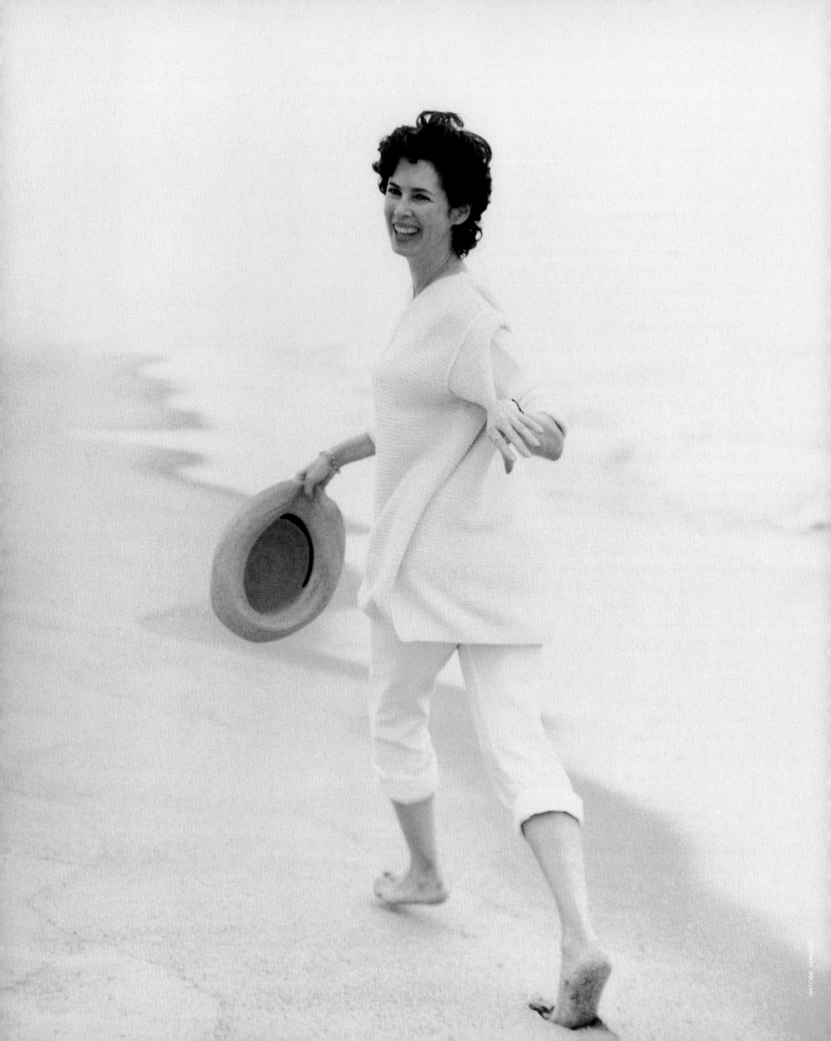

HEADING SOUTH

Isn't it time to reevaluate our definition of a great body? There is no such thing as a perfect body . . . not at twenty, nor at thirty, and, of course, not as we grow older. Even photographs of seventeen-year-old supermodels are retouched by computers. We all have different types of bodies and it's about time we learn to love what we have. A great body is your best body, at whatever age. A great body is your healthy body.

Personally, I don't aim for perfection—and wouldn't even if such a thing existed. As long as I feel that my body is supporting what I want to accomplish, that it is in good shape and optimum health, I feel that I'm on top of my game, and that feeling gives me an edge. I'm probably in better shape today than I've ever been because I don't take my body for granted, as I did in my twenties. Today, I am more in touch with my body, its capacities and limitations; what I can do and what I can't! I have a wonderful sense of victory about the discipline of allotting daily time for my body's maintenance. Also, at this age I know having my body in good shape enables me to do the other things in life I am so much more interested in doing. A fit, strong body supports my lifestyle.

It's important to be realistic, though. I don't want to be locked up in a gym trying to regain a body I didn't even have in my twenties. When you've had a child, irreversible changes take place in your body. And as we get older, gravity does its job, too. Everything starts heading south. One of the reasons we gain weight, and it all sinks floorward, is our tendency to become more sedentary as we age. Unless we stay active, our muscle mass starts wasting away, starting as early as in our mid-twenties. An average of half a pound of muscle is exchanged every year for half a pound of fat—accompanied by that uncomfortable, familiar tightening of our waistbands. Fat doesn't just happen; the pressures of work, family, and overall busyness slow us down. Yet in reality, all we have to do to combat that famous "middle-age spread" is to pare down the calories and pump up the exercise level.

The worst thing for your health is being a couch potato. Roughly 250,000 people die from inactivity-related causes each year. Statistically, a sedentary lifestyle actually falls into the same risky behavior category as smoking cigarettes, driving drunk, or having unprotected sex. When Audrey Manley released the Surgeon General's report on Physical Activity and Health, she confirmed that not exercising could be as bad for us as smoking. Idleness, she concluded, is becoming a public health problem, citing that "more than 60 percent of adults are not physically active on a regular basis." It is clear that our bodies don't wear out from overuse; they grind to a halt from lack of use. And women, in particular, reap the most benefits from getting fit. In 1989, the Journal of the American Medical Association concluded that, while physically fit men are 53 per-

TIP

My secret is to invest in small weights (3 and 5 lbs.) and keep them in sight so I can lift, even for a short time, while I'm watching TV or listening to music. If you tuck your weights away in the closet, it's "out of sight, out of mind." No matter what form of exercise you choose, my advice is to just keep at it on a regular basis. You'll love your new body and it will love you back.

cent less likely to die before their time versus their inactive contemporaries, physically fit women are 98 percent less at risk. Fit women are also sixteen times less likely to die from any form of cancer (compared to men, at only four times) and half as likely to die from breast cancer as unfit women. If that's not a reason to lace up your cross-trainers, I don't know what is.

The antidote to all of this, then, is to keep moving; the old adage, "use it or lose it" couldn't be more true. The world's longest-living woman, Jeanne Calment, who died in 1997 at age 122, rode a bicycle till she was a hundred years old. So forget gold medal Olympian ambitions. It's what you do daily that counts. According to sports scientist Tony Lycholat, "You don't need a structured exercise program to be fit. Impressive cumulative effects can be gained by moving up a gear in everyday life. It's how you use your body each day, minute by minute, that counts in the end."

The easiest way to increase your activity, of course, is by walking. It's pleasurable and it fits into everyone's lifestyle. Remember: this isn't a fitness program we're talking about, it's a fitness lifestyle. At our age, we are deciding how we want to live from now on, improving the quality of our lives. So, make walking a part of what you do for the rest of your life (see Go Take a Walk, p.110). You'll be better off, in the long run, integrating regular activity into your daily life and sustaining it over time, rather than becoming fit enough to run a marathon—and then letting it all slide. My trainer, Sean, tells me, "It's not the amount of exercise you do, it's doing it consistently that makes the difference."

At the same time, be sure to vary your exercise routine (see Break Out from Your Workout, p. 119) because often it's not the body that tires so much as the mind that grows bored with the same workout. Stay active during the day: Don't drive if you can walk, park farther from your destination than usual, and take the stairs instead of the elevator.

On top of this daily upshift of activity, take the time to schedule a regular exercise class, commit to a gym, or do something active that you love (dance, aerobics, tennis, etc.). People often say, "But I get plenty of exercise—I'm always rushing around." That's just not enough. You'll enjoy a completely new wonderful feeling if you stretch, try a yoga class, build strength with weight training, or go for a brisk twenty-minute walk.

As women, another vital reason to incorporate exercise into our lives is to help fend off the debilitating effects of osteoporosis, a disorder in which a dramatic decrease in bone density results in thin, brittle bones and, consequently, increased susceptibility to crippling bone fractures. The bones of the spine, wrist, and hip can become so thin, they may even fracture under their own weight. Often, these disabling fractures can never be repaired.

Although osteoporosis makes its most rapid assault on one's bone mass between the ages of fifty and sixty-five, all women begin a gradual decline in bone mass around age thirty-five. By incorporating "anti-osteoporosis" lifestyle habits, including sufficient calcium intake (see Vital Vitamins, p. 137) and regular exercise, however, a woman may prevent osteoporosis from developing, or at the very least, reduce her chances of suffering from its incapacitating effects.

TIP

Anyone who's anxious about whether she's vulnerable to osteoporosis can get a bone check. (At particular risk are women with family histories of osteoporosis, or those who drink or smoke heavily.) The most accurate test is called dual energy X-ray absorptiometry (a.k.a. DEXA), and will cost you anywhere between $100 to $250. Most hospitals have these machines, and your doctor can easily refer you.

According to research, the bone density of women who exercise regularly is 5 to10 percent higher than that of sedentary women. Walking, jogging, dancing, and lifting weights are forms of osteoporosis-defying exercises, because in each of these activities, weight is placed on the bones, encouraging the bone cells to build themselves up. (This is why they are known as "weight-bearing exercises.") The body areas most vulnerable to osteoporosis include the hips and the vertebrae in the lower and midback. The minimum recommended workout time to fend off the effects of osteoporosis is between a half hour to a full hour, three to four times a week.

The good news is that when it comes to achieving or boosting fitness, it's never too late to start. Even women who start lifting weights at sixty and seventy see dramatic improvements in muscle strength. The bottom line is that we constantly hear scientists telling us we have the possibility to live longer than ever before. So now, each one of us has to decide: *How* do we want to spend those years? Do we crawl off into the sunset—or do we stride, prance, or leap!

HEADING SOUTH—THE FACTS   Research shows us that the biggest gains in health are made by transforming a sedentary lifestyle into a moderately active one. There are even more, but less dramatic, improvements when an already active lifestyle shifts up another gear. Dr. Steven Blair of the Cooper Institute for Aerobics Research in Dallas studied 13,000 individuals who visited the institute for a health checkup. The patients were grouped according to fitness level—and then followed for eight years. The study showed an obvious link between fitness levels and the number of deaths within the groups. Perhaps predictably, the greatest number of deaths occurred in the group that did absolutely no exercise at all; progressively increased fitness positively correlated with progressively increasing life spans. The greatest difference in survival rate was between the groups that did zero exercise and those that did just "a little." Exercise is one area in life where a little yields a lot . . . so the time to start is now.

It should be encouraging to us all that even a brisk walk of thirty minutes each day dramatically reduces our risk of cardiovascular ailments, arthritis, diabetes, osteoporosis, and some cancers. So what are you sitting around for?

"BEAUTY IS TRUTH,
TRUTH BEAUTY, THAT IS ALL . . .
AND ALL YOU NEED
TO KNOW"

JOHN KEATS

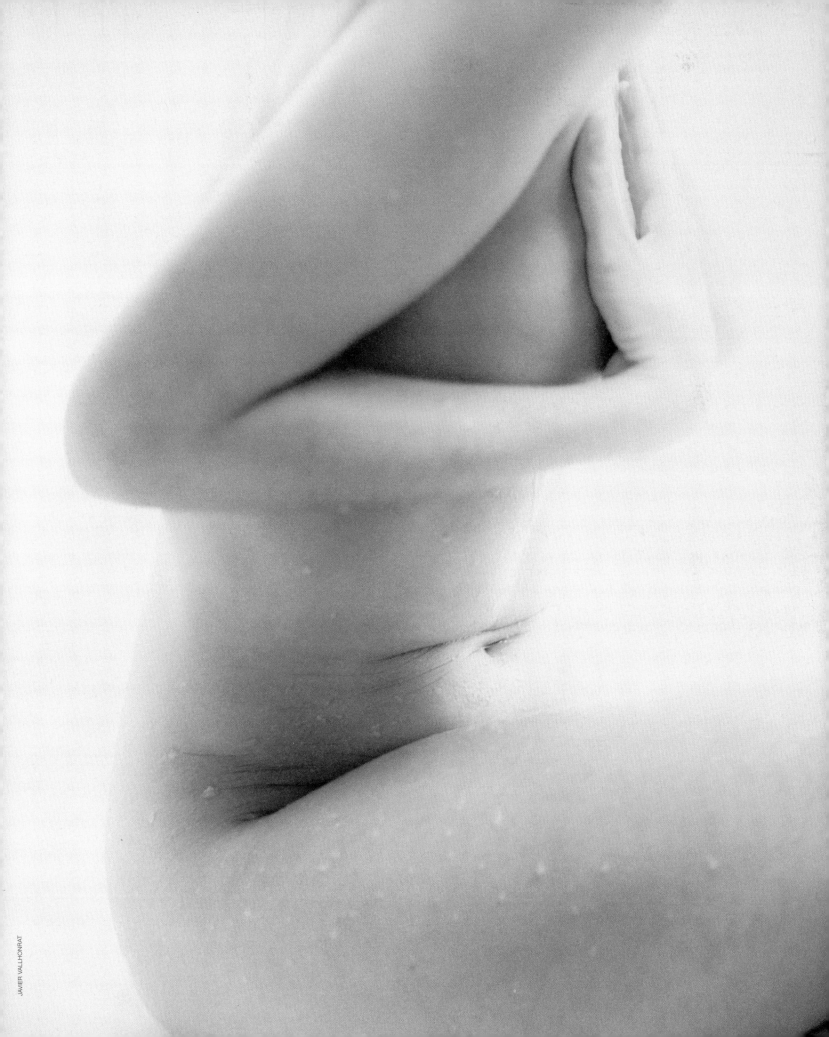

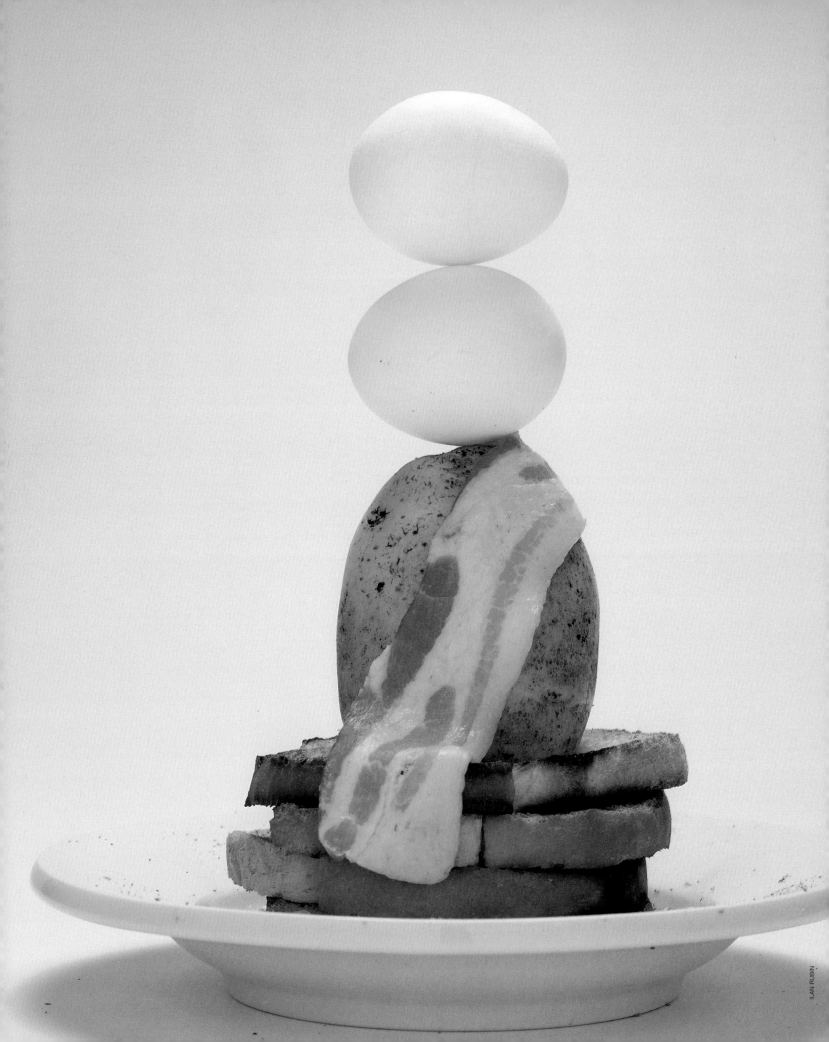

PROBLEM ZONES
THE FIXES . . .

Most of us have an area of the body that we really don't like—and which makes us feel self-conscious. (Almost definitely more than one area!) We all need to realize that millions of other women feel the same about their less-than-perfect parts. I can't think of anyone—not even the world's most gorgeous models—who wouldn't change something if they could.

We should try to let go of the angst of the past and lovingly accept ourselves today. But this doesn't mean there isn't anything we can do about our problem zones. Almost every area of the body, with a little bit of effort and a positive can-do attitude, can be improved. So—here's a head-to-toe self-improvement course: the little fixes that can make a big difference in how you look and, most important, in how you feel.

CELLULITE   The truth is that almost every women ends up with at least a little cellulite after age thirty. (When our skin begins to naturally lose its resilience, the interconnective tissue between our skin and muscles starts to stretch, and the middle-age spread starts to settle in.) Genes also play a part here: If your mother (or your sister) has cellulite, chances are you probably do, too. But the other truth is that cellulite is ordinary fat, which can therefore be managed with diet and exercise. This is where discipline and a little extra effort has a payoff. To help flush toxins from the system: exercise, stretch, walk briskly, eat healthy foods, and drink plenty of water. Simply boosting the circulation can have a positive effect.

Diet can be a big factor in cellulite buildup. Sugary, fatty foods are culprits, and so is skipping meals; when your body doesn't know when the next square meal is coming, it stores fat. Cellulite may be linked to a diet that's full of processed foods, which don't always provide sufficient nutrients. We should be eating fresh fruit, vegetables, nuts, legumes (beans), fish, and meat.

When we're not getting enough nutrients through our diet, we may also suffer a deficiency in certain trace elements: zinc, nickel, and chromium. This, in turn, can lead to a sugar craving, and that piles on the pounds. So you may want to look at a supplement that features the RDA of these elements (see Vital Vitamins, p. 137). In addition, if you're not getting enough fresh fruit and vegetables, this can interfere with the sodium/potassium balance, which in turn contributes to cellulite. Avoid caffeinated drinks, too, which encourage water retention as, of course, does salt.

Try to eat foods that are as pure as possible—without additives, colorings, flavorings, artificial sweeteners, or pesticides. One theory holds that the body can't cope with these chemicals—so it wraps them in fat and stores them on the hips and thighs! Body brushing, as I've explained in Body Care, p. 88, is another technique that many women swear by for conquering cellulite.

TIP

I believe that cellulite creams can do some good; although they aren't miracle workers, some of them contain a caffeine-cola ingredient that boosts circulation. The very action of massaging them into skin helps keep the blood flowing.

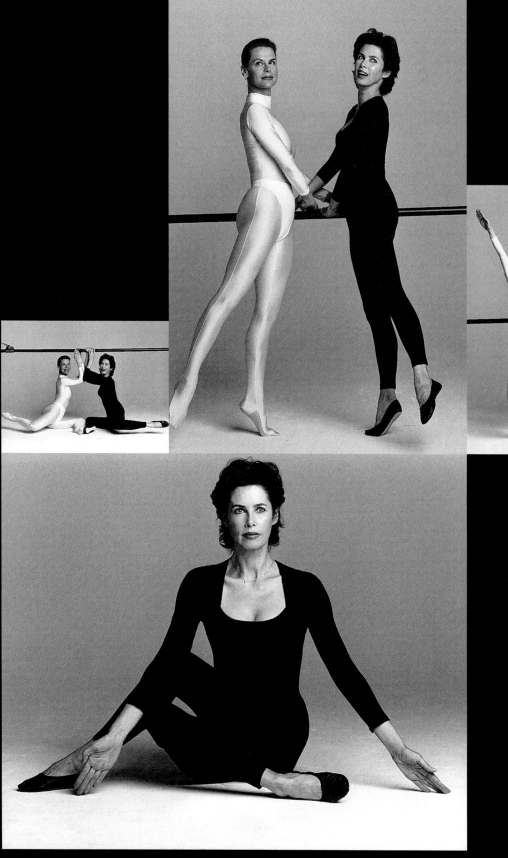

ROUGH HEELS   First, prepare skin: Exfoliated skin absorbs moisture more efficiently. Use a pumice stone or a foot file (from the drugstore) on wet feet to rub away the built-up skin. (I don't believe in using a blade to cut the skin.) Then dry your feet and apply your heaviest, most moisturizing hand cream. Neutrogena Norwegian Formula Hand Cream can really help here. In tests it soothed and healed coal miners' bleeding hands, so it can certainly tackle our rough heels and the hard pads under our toes! The luxury of an occasional pedicure will clear away a lot of dead skin, making it easier for you to keep up the great results at home. Be conscious, too, that if your shoe rubs against your foot, it can lead to hard skin buildup; pad your shoes with Band-Aids or special shoe pads that you can find at the drugstore.

SCALY ELBOWS   The effect of a woman dressed to the nines can be spoiled immediately by dry, scaly, even dirty-looking elbows. Elbows have almost no oil glands, so they can get parched very quickly, especially as we get older and oil production slows down. If you tend to rest your elbows on flat surfaces, it only aggravates the problem; even your clothes can strip oils from the skin. I like to add as much moisture as I can to this area; if I'm applying hand cream, I'll be sure to extend it right on up to my elbows, and I regularly scrub them with a little brush to stop them from drying out. (It's best to brush your elbows in the shower or after you bathe, while the skin is still moist.)

DROOPY KNEES   Knees, like heels, tend to get super dry. The solution: Slather on moisture. But for gravity-reversal, you'll need to exercise. Walking is wonderful for the knees. Lotte Berk (see Break Out from Your Workout, p. 119) has a tremendous exercise that tightens the whole knee area.

PLIÉ   (Use a heavy chair for support)

1   Stand with heels together, making a 45-degree angle with your feet.
2   Raise heels two inches.
3   Pull in abdominal muscles.
4   Bend knees and lower torso two inches; raise right arm and lift back.
5   Keep abs taut and shoulders down. Lower and lift ten times.
6   Shake out legs. Repeat twice.

TIP

If your elbows are really dingy and need "bleaching," try this trick: cut a lemon in half and rest with your elbows cupped in the lemon halves for ten to fifteen minutes. Then rinse and apply a rich moisturizer. It works wonders.

REAR END HEADING SOUTH
Only exercise can reverse this unfortunate descent. At Lotte Berk they place a special emphasis on exercises for the rear. I find these two to be *very* effective.

FANNY LIFT

1 Stand behind a backward facing chair, supporting your hands on the back.
2 Stand tall with your feet together.
3 Extend your right leg back with your foot pointed.
4 Rise up on the ball of your left foot, keeping both legs straight, pelvis tucked in.
5 Holding the tuck, lift your right leg behind you about two inches then lower two inches, as shown.
6 Lift and lower thirty times. Shake out right leg.
7 Repeat once more from the beginning, still working your right leg. Switch legs; repeat twice.

PRETZEL

(This works the waist and back muscles, as well as the buttocks)
1 Sit with your right leg bent, in front of the body, left leg back.
2 Rotate left hip forward so that left foot rises.
3 Lift left knee twenty times, keeping hips forward, shoulders down. Repeat. Switch leg positions; repeat sequence twice.

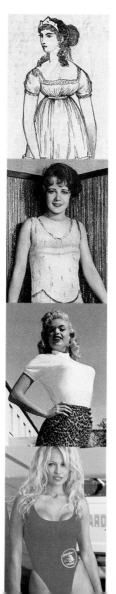

BUST BOOSTERS
The really quick, low-cost, absolutely best way to lift breasts that aren't as pert as they used to be is a good bra! We have manipulated our breasts throughout history: forcing them upward in the Empire period, flattening them during the Flapper era, and turning them into ice-cream cones in the '50s! Breasts have been out and breasts have been in. Today, you can have the bust shape you want—with everything from an oomph-giving Wonderbra to a minimizer. For me, the best shape is fairly natural and round—but higher does look younger; sometimes all it takes is hiking up those straps a little. Spend an afternoon bra shopping.

Of course, you can strengthen the underlying chest muscles with those "I-must-I-must-increase-my-bust" exercises we all did in high school: Place the heels of your hands together, push, and release. Repeat as often (and as frequently) as you want—but don't expect miracles.

GOOD OLD PUSH UPS
. . . but from the knees. Work up to three sets of ten.

CHEST PRESS

1   Lie on your back, with your legs bent, feet on the floor, tummy muscles pulled in fairly tight, and arms out to either side.

2   Bend your arms upward at the elbow (almost as if you are surrendering!).

3   Now, with fists closed, bring your arms together until elbows and fore arms meet above your chest. Create resistance to feel your chest and arm muscles working.

4   Lower to the starting point and repeat fifteen times.

5   As your muscles strengthen, add light hand weights.

What makes breasts look saggy and unattractive is the crepiness that age and yo-yo dieting can bring. Also, after pregnancy, the breasts can lose their elasticity. We tend to neglect our breasts, but it's important to lavish creams on this delicate area. I don't believe that special "bust creams" really make any difference—but I moisturize all over with my regular body cream on a daily basis. (Like the elbows, the breast area has few oil glands, and so is prone to dryness). When I was pregnant, I religiously applied a rich, lanolin cream to all the areas that might develop stretch marks (including my hips). And it worked! I didn't develop a single mark. Even if you did get stretch marks, over the years, moisturizing the breasts can minimize the visibility of those silvery lines. Of course, there are many other reasons we may have stretch marks; birth control pills, menopause, or dramatic weight swings can all trigger these marks. And, as with most body dynamics, some of us are simply more susceptible to them than others.

FLABBY ARMS

Flabby underarms are tremendously aging. (We've all waved good-bye to someone—and been mortified to see our underarms flapping away in the wind! I believe some could even create dangerous wind patterns!) These are my time-tested exercises that firm up this troublesome area, fast. And, the best news is that you can do these exercises at your desk or while watching TV or any time you've got a few extra minutes for yourself.

WEIGHTS FOR ARMS

Here's another exercise that's great for the arms.

1   With a two- or three-pound weight in your left hand, step forward on the right leg (opposite leg and hand).

2   Bend your right knee, straightening the left leg behind you.

3   Lean your weight over the bent right knee and keep your back in a straight line.

4   With weight in hand, raise your left arm straight back behind you.

5   Make tiny movements, lifting in toward the body and up. Do about thirty on each arm.

ROUNDED TUMMY This is a tough one. Women naturally have a slightly Marilyn Monroe-shaped belly, and it's hard to defy nature. This gets worse in middle age—the classic "spread"—and scientists are now discovering why. One group of European scientists discovered that the enzyme lipoprotein lipase (which is responsible for the growth of fat cells), becomes more active in abdominal cells than in other regions of the body as women pass through menopause and estrogen levels plummet. So more fat is deposited around the middle than other areas. All-over aerobic exercise, like brisk walking, will help because it burns calories. Lotte Berk and Pilates can spot-target the stomach area, but these exercises really need to be supervised. Done incorrectly, abdominal exercises—in particular crunches—can develop the muscles so that the tummy actually protrudes even more than it did before. So proceed carefully.

In the old days, we used to do crunches by hooking our feet under a heavy object and curling up. Exercise professionals believe there's a much better way. This will prevent back and neck problems, which can also result if crunches are performed improperly, and ensure that you get the maximum tummy-tightening benefit.

1   Lie on the floor with your knees bent, hip-width apart, soles of the feet flat on the floor.
2   Place your hands behind your head—but don't lace your fingers together. Your chin should be about a fist's distance from your chest.
3   Curl slowly upward, in a controlled movement—don't jerk. You want to avoid stiffly lifting your torso off the floor; instead, aim to lift one vertebra off the floor at a time, using the power of your abdominal muscles.
4   Keep your head, neck, and arms frozen in the same position. Don't use your hands to push your head forward; instead, it is better for your neck if you press back gently into your hands with your head. Your head, neck, and arms play no part in lifting you off the floor; your abdominal muscles should be doing all the work. Yanking your head is one reason why some people complain that crunches (literally) give them a pain in the neck.
5   As you curl, tighten your abdominal muscles and then breathe out forcefully through your mouth. As you lower yourself down again slowly—and in a controlled way—keep your abdominal muscles tight and inhale through your nose.

How you can tell if you're in the right position: When you do a crunch, freeze-frame at the top of the movement. You should not be able to draw a straight line through the part of your back that's lifted off the floor; instead, your torso should be in a slightly rounded, almost C-shaped position.

BODYSHAPES

Understanding your natural body shape enables you to be realistic about what you can and can't achieve. By our middle years, we should all have a handle on our basic body type—where the fat piles on and where it comes off quickly. It's completely unrealistic to open up a magazine, look at a beautiful body, and compare yourself. Unless your last name is Crawford or Schiffer, you'll likely end up feeling depressed and defeated by what you see. I've said it before and I'll say it again: Even the models don't really have the bodies you see in the magazines. One particular supermodel was "stretched" by a computer for a Cosmo magazine cover that had the whole fashion industry talking—because in real life, even her fabulous body wasn't quite the perfection that was glorified on the cover.

When it comes to body shape, we basically have to make do with what nature—and our genes—gave us. I believe that many body types can be beautiful and I celebrate our differences. My friend Elizabeth has a body that's voluptuous and round and completely beautiful; she certainly doesn't look like most images you'd find in a magazine. But she has her own look and shape, and it is fabulous. (What's more, men love it!) So it isn't all about being thin. The test I use to determine what kind of shape I am in is not how much I weigh, but how good I feel in my clothes.

It's certainly true, though, that as we age, we tend to accumulate extra fat around our middle—part of that midage hormone havoc! But it is possible to turn your waist and hips into a no-parking zone for fat. The key to staying trim and shapely forever is to pare down your calories and rev up your activity. If you choose activities that are most suited to your particular body type (see Shape Shifting, p.107), then you really can help your body fend off unwanted fat. So in this case, it's use it . . . and lose it!

Any exercise that is aerobic and gets the metabolism going will burn both calories and fat. Walking is probably the ultimate all-over fat burner, but it really helps those problem hips and thighs as well. One of the toughest places to trim and tone is the upper arms (see Problem Zones—The Fixes, p. 99). I have found the Lotte Berk and Pilates methods (see Break Out from Your Workout, p. 119) help spot-target problem areas, because they concentrate on isolating and working individual muscles. My experience is that these two types of exercise help to create a natural body "girdle" by intensely working the muscles, which then hold everything in.

So get off your butt and get active! Use the stairs whenever you can. You use different muscle groups going up and down stairs, so be sure to do both. Park the car farther away from the store than usual and walk the rest of the way. Pop in a favorite tape, turn up the volume, and attack your household chores. You have to do them anyway, so why not get the added bonus of burning extra calories and enjoying yourself? Gardening is a great activity for the waist and leg muscles; bend, stretch, reach, and squat. Walk, walk, walk, walk, walk; break up your day with walks. Stretch and tone with rubber Dyna-Bands (see Resources). Sex can be great exercise, too! It can be a terrific calorie-burner—and a wonderful circulation booster.

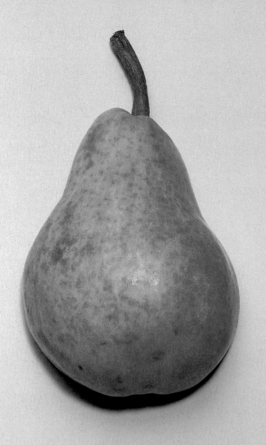
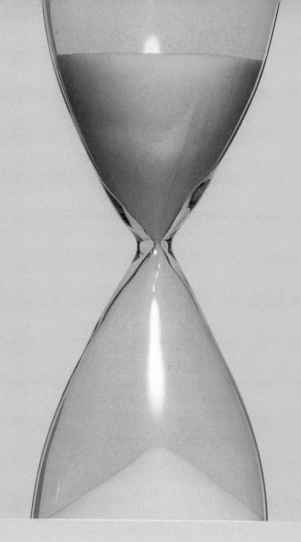
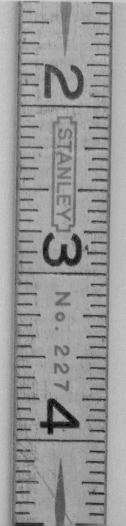
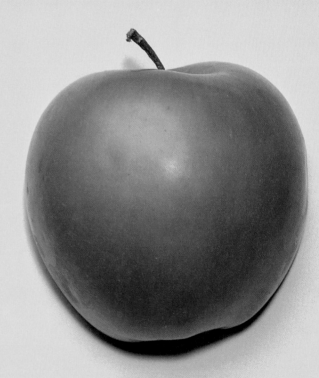

SHAPE SHIFTING   Identifying your body shape will enable you to choose the best exercises for you. If you choose the wrong exercises, you may end up building up muscle in undesirable places. The StairMaster may be great for you, but your best friend may end up with bulky calves if she does the same routine. Everything in moderation is fine, but certain exercise workouts can overdevelop some areas quickly.

Yoga and the methods based on stretching of Pilates and Lotte Berk, are suitable for all body types and perfect for all-over toning and firming. But if you want to break out from your normal workout, here are some targeted body-type inspirations to try:

APPLE SHAPED

ARE YOU APPLE SHAPED, WITH A FULLER UPPER BODY, ROUNDED MIDDLE AND NARROW/SLIM HIPS?

• Choose activities that tone your upper body, trim down your waist, and build up your legs and buttocks: walking, cycling, hill-climbing, step classes (which will also help reduce fat deposits in the upper back and bust), crunches, arm curls
• It's best to avoid: swimming, rowing, or exercises for the upper part of the body that involve weights

PEAR SHAPED

ARE YOU PEAR-SHAPED, WITH SMALLER SHOULDERS, WIDER HIPS, AND HEAVIER LEGS?

• Try activities that tone and trim your legs, thighs, and buttocks and build up your shoulders: swimming, rowing, canoeing, walking, bicycling long distances on flat surfaces, DynaBands or light weight workouts, playing tennis, low-intensity aeorobics
• Try to avoid: stair climbing, which builds muscles in the butt and thighs, step classes, bicycling up hills or mountains

HOURGLASS SHAPED

ARE YOU CURVY, WITH A CLASSIC HOURGLASS SHAPE?

• Seek out activities that work your top and bottom halves and use only moderate weights: swimming, volleyball, cross-country skiing, walking, biking, running
• Stay away from: stair climbing, heavy weight training
• Try to vary your routine as much as possible, so that you work the whole body evenly.

RULER SHAPED

ARE YOU STRAIGHT UP AND DOWN—LIKE A RULER?

• Look for exercises that add shapeliness and curves, particularly around your waist, buttocks and shoulder areas: boxing, swimming, circuit-training, rowing, skating, calisthenics classes. Hiking, biking, and yoga are good bets, too.

EXERCISE

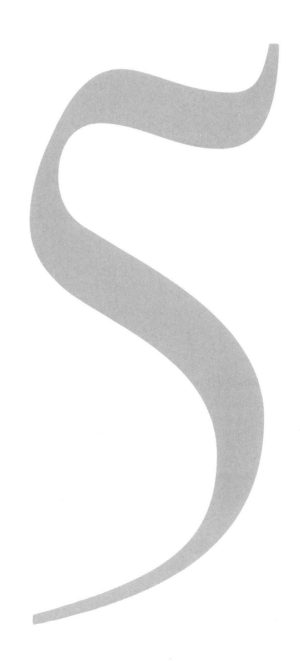

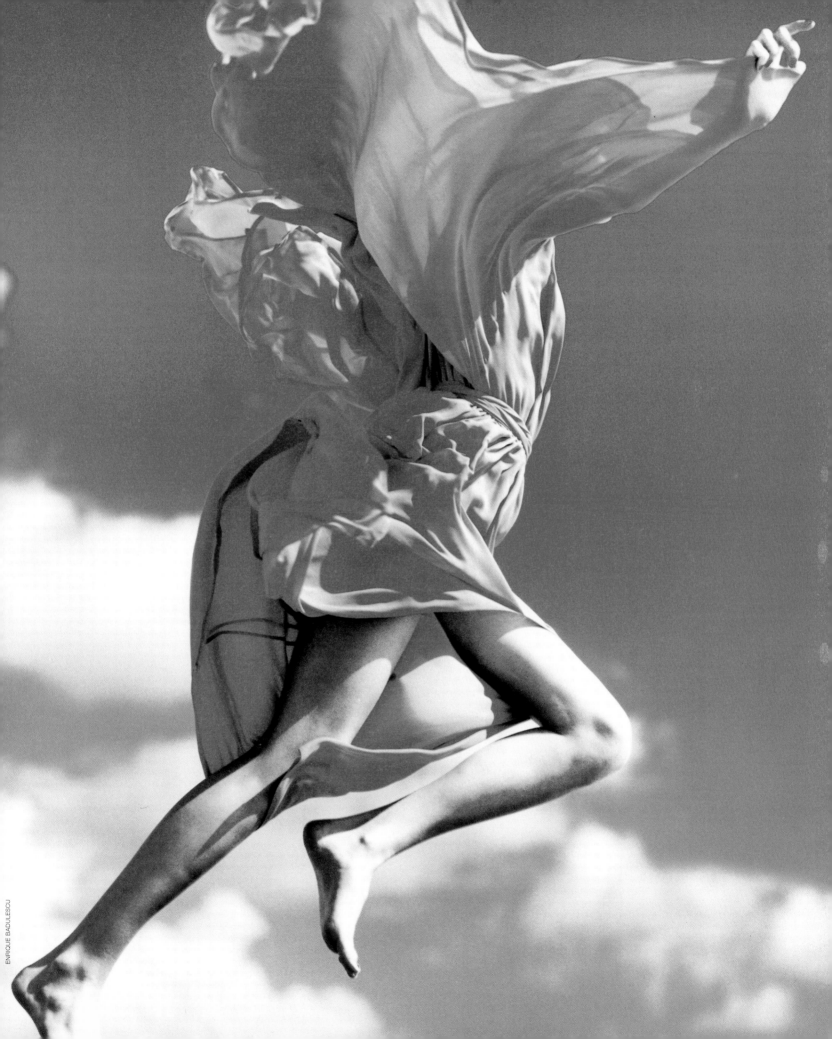

GO TAKE A WALK

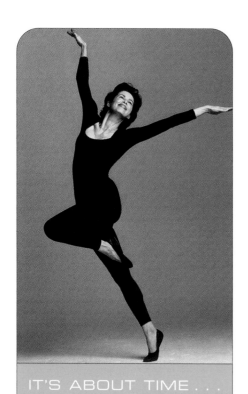

IT'S ABOUT TIME . . .

Hippocrates called walking "man's best medicine." Well, it's woman's, too. At a certain age, most of us reach a point where we have tried just about every exercise going: We've experimented with aerobics, signed up for one-on-one training, or invested in equipment that is probably gathering dust in the spare bedroom! Well, maybe you have to reach a certain age to appreciate that the ultimate exercise doesn't require special clothes or machines or appointments or a gym membership. It is completely portable, very easy, and doesn't cost a dime. All you need is a comfortable pair of shoes.

At the very least, walking is a two-for-one exercise for me. Regular, normal-paced walking keeps the weight at bay and is the easiest, simplest way to calm the mind and get a new perspective on the ups and downs of life. There is really no excuse for not doing it; and, if you make walking a habit, it's something you can do into your sixties, seventies, eighties, nineties! Because, unlike almost every other exercise you've tried, walking is the one you'll never give up.

It is also a sanity saver. Every thirty minutes I spend walking feels like I've just added sixty bonus minutes to my day. If you just take the time for a walk, it will feel like you have more time (and energy!) to tackle what you have to do afterward. (If you don't believe me, just try it.) We live so much inside our heads, sometimes we actually need the change of pace to change our mindset. What seemed so important before a walk—a problem, a deadline, an energy vacuum—suddenly seems so much more manageable afterward; stepping outside gives us a better perspective on what it is we're trying to achieve.

I have different kinds of walks. There's my Madison Avenue, peppy, non-stop A-to-B walk. (My trainer, Sean, reminds me: If I want to count this as a workout, window shopping is not allowed!) Or, there's my morning stroll through Central Park. It sets me up for the rest of the day—in the peace before the world gets up, when the day and the early morning serenity still belong to me. And finally, I often enjoy my invigorating evening trek: the lights, crisp air, and moonlit skyline are a beautiful end to any day. In a new city, I find walking is the greatest way to explore and truly experience a new place. Also, I've found that a brisk walk after a long flight is the greatest jet-lag cure of all. Just as with the Magic Bath (see p.150), find what and when works best for you—so you can prescribe the perfect walk for that moment.

It's great fun to walk with a friend. You encourage each other and when one of you doesn't feel up to it, you always have the other to make sure the deal is kept. Just don't walk to the ice-cream parlor!

The secret, I've found, is to walk regularly. Exercise pros generally prescribe thirty minutes, at least four times a week, at a brisk pace. There's no need to speed walk. You shouldn't feel exhausted at the end. Regular, casual-pace walking really keeps the weight off. My friend Michele had a problem with her weight since childhood, until we started our regular walks together. Making very

... to have a fit, healthy body that will support what we want to achieve in years to come. That doesn't mean running a marathon: It means upping our activity levels and getting off the couch, so that we can defy not only time, but gravity. For me, the secret is gentle, regular exercise. It's a way of living—and moving—that boosts your energy level and calms your mind. It works for me—and it can work for you.

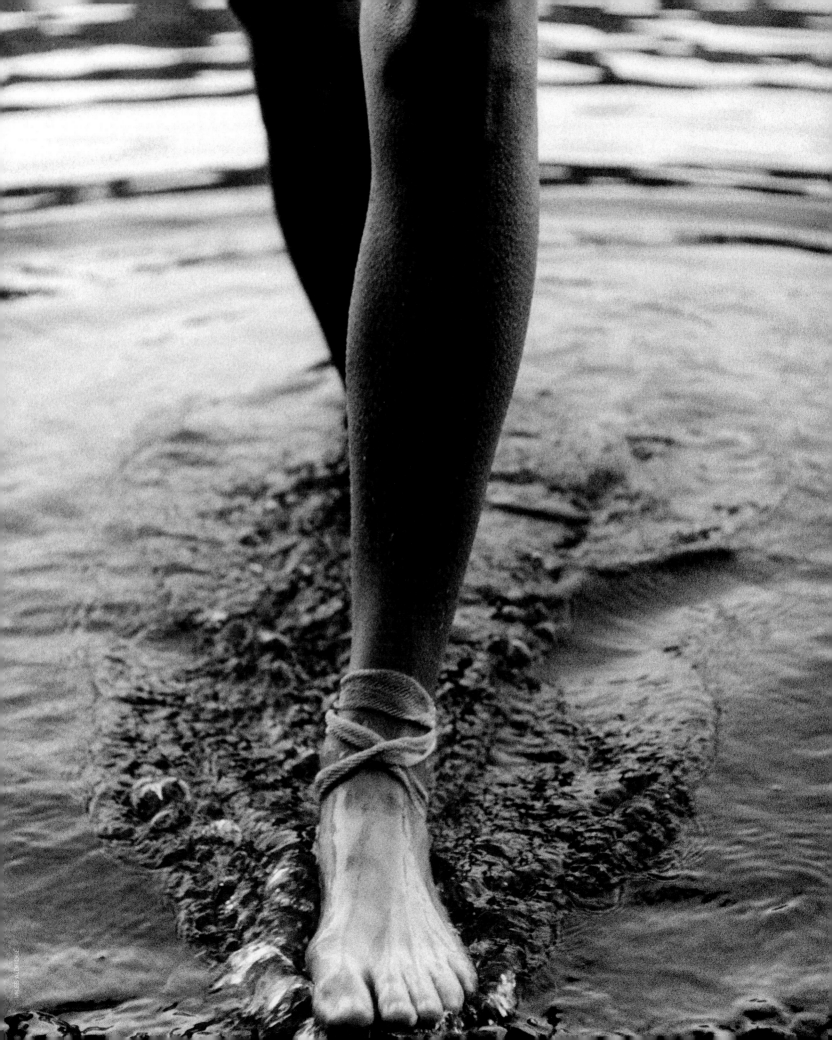

few changes in her diet, just walking every day, Michele not only lost weight, but now effortlessly keeps it off and feels fantastic. The key is simply to start, and to take it one day at a time. But I promise, in as little time as a week, you'll see and feel a difference.

WALKING WISDOM

• Comfortable feet make you look beautiful. Really! Because if something's tough on your feet, it will definitely show on your face. In New York, I tend to wear flat shoes during the day, because I love walking whenever I can. I save the high heels for night. (If you need to wear elegant shoes where you're heading, throw them in a tote and put them on when you arrive.)

• As far as I'm concerned, Dr. Scholl is the patron saint of walkers. In pharmacies and footwear stores, check out anything that might make walking more comfortable for you: inner soles (for extra cushioning), corn pads, heel grips, whatever. Trust me. One blister will ruin the whole experience.

• Be prepared for all the great ideas you'll have while you're walking. I use walking for dreaming, problem solving, and meditating. Buckminster Fuller, architect, engineer, inventor, and poet, known as one of the most original thinkers of the twentieth century, said that when we have an idea, we have eleven seconds to get it down before it disappears; don't kid yourself you're going to remember that amazing brainwave when you get home. Places like The Sharper Image and many catalogs often carry little "Voice-It" recorders—credit card–sized gizmos that you can carry in your pocket to vocally record your ideas at the touch of a button. (I have a great one made by Sony—see Resources.)

• Aerobic slouch socks are great for walking: try to find a pair that's double thick at the heel and ball of your foot (cushioning, again). When you're shopping for socks and tights, avoid anything with a seam across the toes or on the side of your foot; as you walk, that little seam starts to feel like a great big log in your shoe and it can become agonizing.

• Carry the right bag: a shoulder bag throws your posture out and can cause back trouble. I like little waist packs that clip around like a belt and allow me to keep my hands free. Or if I need a little more room, I love a back pack. It keeps any weight I'm carrying balanced, so I can really walk! (You can find them at every price level, from Gap to Gucci.) If you have to carry a shoulder bag, make it a lightweight nylon one and wear it diagonally across your chest, switching shoulders often.

• Wear a hat in winter to keep in the warmth and in summer to keep off the sun. Don't forget sun protection—not just on your face, but on your hands, as well.

• Drink water before, during, and after your walk. Drink a little extra in warm weather and avoid walking during the hottest hours.

• Be a Girl Scout, always prepared: keep Kleenex in your pocket for that runny nose on cold days and be sure to dress in layers. You may be freezing when you first step outside, but you'll feel like you're having a hot flash minutes later, and you'll want to be able to peel off layers, tying them round your waist. And don't forget gloves, if you think you'll need them.

• Music, on a Walkman, can help your walking workout. I find I walk a little faster and a bit farther when I've got my tape on. Experiment and find out what revs you up!

WALK THIS WAY... According to the World Health Organization, the gentle art of walking delivers a range of health benefits, helping lower blood pressure and cholesterol levels, improving strength, strengthening bones, and building stamina—and of course, boosting our mood and energy level. A regular walking program is also one of the best ways to protect yourself both from the common cold and more serious illnesses: In a study of two groups of women in their thirties and forties, researchers had one group stick to their usual couch potato lifestyle while the other group walked for forty-five minutes, five days a week. The walkers reported half as many days with flu or cold symptoms as the nonwalkers, and their antibody levels (which help fight infection), rose steadily during the fifteen-week study.

Try to walk every day, increasing your distance until you're moving at a steady pace for twenty to sixty minutes. If you're really out of condition, start with just five or ten minutes and you should find that within six to eight weeks, you'll work up to the optimum workout: thirty to forty minutes at least four times a week. Swinging your arms vigorously (in opposition to your leg movements) can help you burn 5 to 10 percent more calories, and so will accelerating your speed; walking at 2.5 miles per hour (a twenty-four-minute mile) for thirty minutes expends 105 calories, while at 4.5 miles per hour (just over a thirteen-minute mile), you'll burn off 200 calories. And try to vary your terrain; unsurprisingly, climbing hills uses more calories—as does walking on sand, gravel, or grass. But even a leisurely stroll is infinitely better than no exercise at all. With walking, you win on so many levels, so . . . *Go take a hike!*

S-T-R-E-T-C-H

If a door isn't opened and closed regularly, it becomes creaky and rusty. That's roughly what happens to your joints if you don't move them regularly. Moving and stretching is something you can do at any time of the day, almost anywhere—with an instant payback! You get a feeling of energy and oxygen rushing through the body. Stretching "unkinks" muscles and busts stress; our muscles tense up and clench during the day and anything that helps release those blockages is good for us. Stretching also has an aesthetic benefit. It actually helps prevent muscles from getting too bulky, creating a sleeker, more elongated body. When I was training with the Canadian Ballet Company, Les Grands Ballet Canadiens, we would alternate every muscle-building exercise with a muscle-*stretching* exercise to ensure long, elegant, yet muscled silhouettes. And besides, stretching just *feels* great!

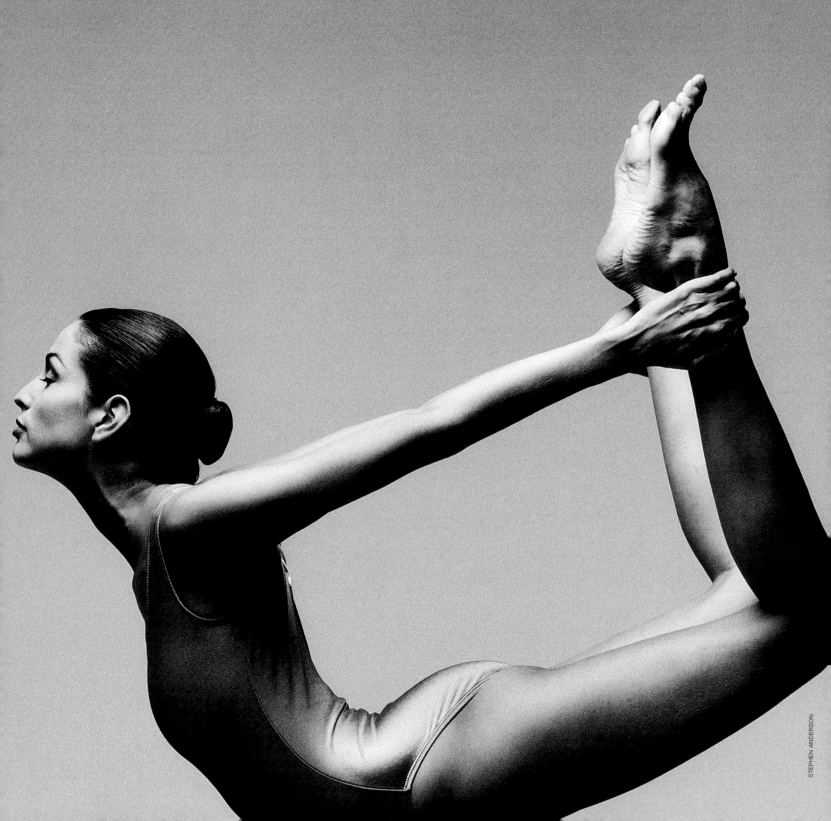

"IF ONE IS OUT OF TOUCH WITH ONESELF,
THEN ONE CANNOT TOUCH OTHERS"

ANNE MORROW LINDBERGH

STEPHEN ANDERSON

The older we get, the more important it is for us to stretch. I've noticed many older people as they walk down the street—hunched over, stiff, and con-stricted—having lost that loose-limbed freedom and flexibility of youth. This "seizing-up" of the body immediately announces, "I'm old": Time has done its work, and age has set in almost *because* of the lack of flexibility. I don't care if you're wearing the greatest dress or have the best new hairdo; if you're stiff and not at ease with your body, you'll definitely look older. With daily stretching, you can hang onto that youthful flexibility for a lifetime. And if you make it a part of your life—like brushing your teeth or combing your hair—it will become one of your best anti-aging secrets. What's more, by combating stiffness, staying limber actually helps prevent falls—a serious hazard to women as we get older.

Stretching also strengthens muscles. As flexibility increases, so does your muscle power; you're able to generate more force because the muscle is in a lengthened position. The right stretches give flexibility and support to the back and neck, too. I hear so many friends complain of back problems, but stretching can *really* help here. You might say, "I don't have the time to stretch"—yet Americans lose millions of work days a year because of bad backs. Stretching is like the "stitch-in-time-saves-nine" philosophy. (Or in this case, a "stretch in time saves you to ninety-nine!")

EASY STRETCHES

SHOULDER RELEASE

Sit back on your heels. (If this is hard on the knees, put a little cushion between your legs, your rear, and under your knees.) Clasp your hands behind your back and move your upper body forward until your forehead is touching the floor. Keeping your hands clasped, raise them toward your head and hold them there. Let your arms hang and relax. (You can also do this stretch standing up.)

HIP PRESS

Place your hands firmly on a table in front of you, shoulder-width apart. Step back from the table. Bend one knee, lift the other leg, and cross it over the knee. Sit back into the hip. Reverse and repeat.

THE YOGA "COBRA" STRETCH

Lie full length, flat on your stomach, ankles slightly apart. Bend your arms and place the palms of your hands flat on the ground underneath your shoulders. Slowly push upward so that the top of your spine lifts off the ground, being careful not to arch. Don't strain the neck, but keep your head in a line with the upper part of your back. Hold the stretch, return to the resting position, and repeat.
NOTE: Beginners, try to keep the palm and forearm on the floor. More advanced stretchers, try to straighten out the arms.

One word of caution: if you force a cold muscle while stretching, you can easily pull it. You should always be very careful to start slowly and gently, never rushing yourself. There's no need to force a stretch; flexibility will come amazingly quickly, if you simply do it on a regular basis.

ARM RELAXER

A great stretch for opening out the shoulders and unkinking tension is to do the arm movements of a yoga exercise called the "Eagle." Place one elbow over the other, straight in front of you. Then snake your arms around each other, with your hands touching palms to fingers in a prayer-like position— almost in line with your eyes. Hold, then reverse.

ADVANCED STRETCHES

As you become more limber (and you will), here are some more challenging stretches. Again, always take it easy—and warm up first.

SPINAL TWIST

Kneel down with your left leg folded under you. Then place the right leg over the left knee, putting the foot flat on the ground. Wrap your right arm around your right knee, twisting around, and placing your hand behind you. Try to look as far as you can over your left shoulder.

"THREADING THE NEEDLE" STRETCH

A variation on one of the simple stretches: Sit back on your heels. Clasp your hands behind your back and move forward until your forehead is touching the floor. Keep the hands clasped and hold the stretch there, then take your right hand and thread it under your left shoulder, twisting your upper body so that your ear is on the ground. Hold. Repeat, threading the left hand under the right shoulder.

THE BUTTERFLY STRETCH

Lie on your back and wrap your knees, one knee in front of the other, keeping them at a 90-degree angle to the ground. Reach forward and gently pull your legs toward you, so that you get a stretch in the back of your thighs and through your hips. Once you've finished (and alternated legs), place your arms flat on the floor and take your top leg over and out to the side, until it is resting on the floor. Turn your head to face in the opposite direction, to deepen the stretch.

LEG SPLIT

Once you're fully warmed up, sit on the floor with your legs in front of you, spread as wide apart as you can comfortably manage. Placing your forearm on the ground on the inside of your thigh for support, look up toward the ceiling and slowly reach over your leg with your opposite arm. Keep your tummy in. Then twist your torso so that it's directly over the leg and lean forward, either with a rounded back or with a flat back. (You get a different kind of stretch with each.) With a rounded back, walk your hands into the middle, between your legs, and straighten your back. Then reach across to your other leg and repeat, starting with the first part of the exercise.

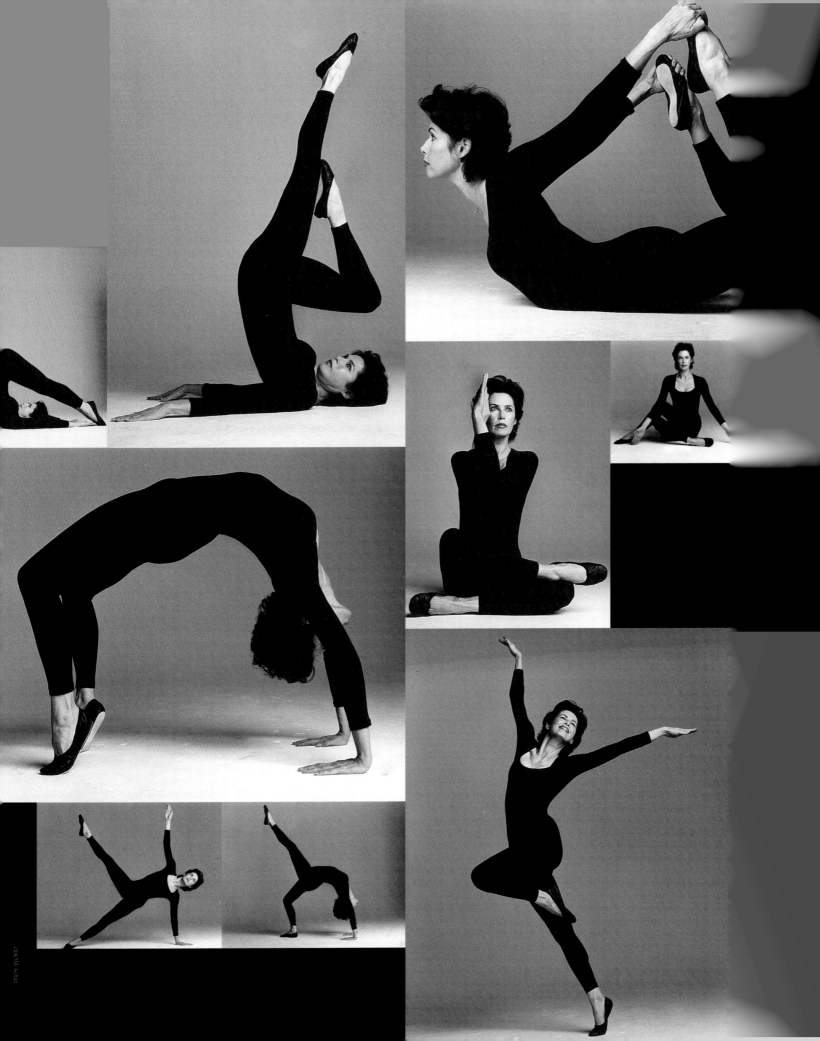

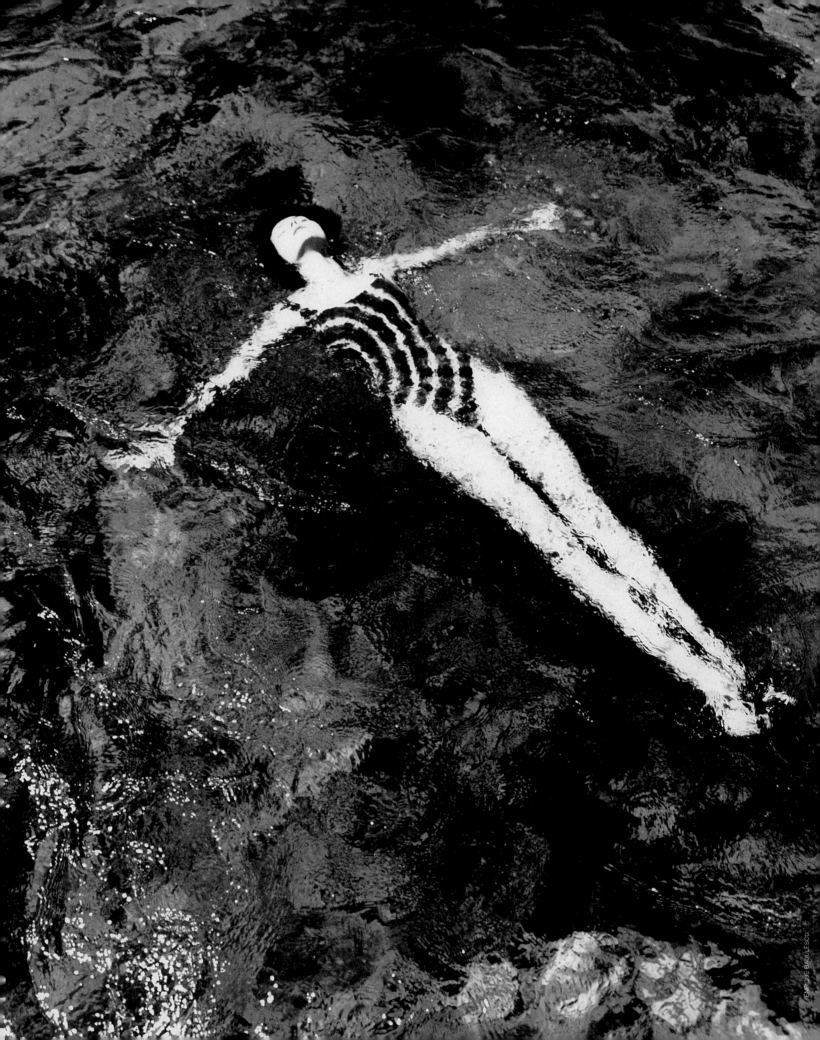

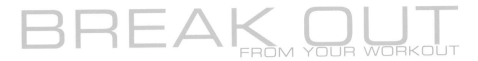

BREAK OUT
FROM YOUR WORKOUT

Almost everyone who exercises regularly gets workout burnout at some point. The sheer boredom of doing the same exercises, week in, week out, can get to you. You have to find ways of varying your workout before the boredom sets in and you crash and burn. Keep it fun. Keep it flexible. Don't look at exercising as something you do only between 6 and 7 P.M. on Monday, Wednesday, and Friday; integrate it into your life and up your activity level all around. Variety is the spice of exercise. (The exercise pros call it "cross-training.")

Try to be creative about activities that keep you moving. Tucked away in the back of my mind, I have the possibility of taking up golf someday, because it will take me outdoors—and it'll continue to keep me off my butt in my later years! If you have the good fortune to go to a spa, you'll be able to experience different kinds of exercises—sample different ways of working out.

Many gyms and sporting goods stores now have a large inflatable gymnastic ball (called a body ball and available in different sizes) to bounce and work out on—which is a lot harder than it looks. Or try a climbing wall or swing on a trapeze. In fact, any circus skills can be a wonderful creative outlet and make you feel like a kid again. At one of the gyms I attend in New York, Drago's, I've watched men and women in their sixties, seventies, and even eighties on parallel bars and the trapeze (see Resources). So be daring!

Try a friend's exercise class. Go rowboating with a child instead of going to the movies. Kick a ball around with a teenager. Take a cross-country skiing vacation. Mow the lawn. (Apparently, pushing a mower burns as many calories as low impact aerobics, tennis, or downhill skiing.) Be creative at finding ways that keep your metabolism fired up, and you will feel uplifted because you haven't forced yourself into anything.

There are three types of exercise, though, that I return to time and again: yoga (you can now find classes throughout the country), the Lotte Berk method, and Pilates. The latter two are decribed below. All of these forms of movement combine the benefits of strength building and silhouette slimming.

T'AI CHI CHUAN This form of exercise is often bracketed with the martial arts, but it's actually more like a moving meditation. The focus is so calming that it completely cuts you off from the day-to-day problems—at least for that moment.

In T'ai Chi (*chi* is Chinese for life force), slow, flowing movements follow a set pattern, enabling you to harmonize mind, body, and spirit and become more deeply centered in yourself. Legend has it that T'ai Chi was originated by Chang Sanfeng, a thirteenth-century Taoist monk, who adapted an earlier martial art form used by the monks for protection. As the story goes, Chang Sanfeng was observing the movements animals make—and saw that they were mostly circular ones. He joined them together to create a set of postures, with almost dance-like movements. The emphasis in doing these movements isn't on strength or exertion, but on concentration, relaxation, and balance. The knees are kept bent and movement is achieved by shifting the greater part of the body's weight slowly from one foot to the other, while the hands make careful and gentle pushing and circling gestures. There's a lot of focus on the correct breathing.

T'ai Chi is often recommended therapeutically for people with tension, anxiety, high blood pressure, and heart complaints because of its relaxing effect. It can promote and maintain good mental and physical health. I have to confess, at the beginning, T'ai Chi can feel maddeningly slow-paced, particularly if you've been used to a strenuous, active workout. In America, we're a very "I-want-it-now" society, but once you get used to T'ai Chi's pace, you'll find it's wonderfully energizing and calming (see suggested reading list).

PILATES   As mentioned earlier, this is one of the best all-round exercise techniques I've ever encountered, virtually burnout-proof and wonderfully rejuvenating, delivering flexibility and strength without bulking up your muscles. It's not sweaty at all—and because so many of the movements work on strengthening the abdomen, it's terrific for bad backs. (The tummy muscles support the back and any flabbiness there is blamed for a lot of back problems.) German-born Joseph Pilates created the technique earlier this century, initially to combat his personal health problems.

Today, using his regimen of precisely controlled movements, Pilates's technique can help you spot-target problem areas in an extraordinarily specific way. You can say, "I hate my saddlebags thighs," and will be given exercises to zone in on that area. Half the class is performed on specially designed equipment using springs and your own body weight; the other half is continued on the mat.

Pilates is also really popular with dancers and injured athletes, because the gentle exercises are so strengthening. Pilates studios—which are now opening in many towns and cities—offer one-on-one instruction, or what they call "mat work" classes, which include several people; you can also do the mat work exercises at home. For more information about Pilates, see Resources.

LOTTE BERK   A German dancer invented it, but it was Lydia Bach, an American, who revised the exercises and brought the method to the United States in 1970: a hybrid of modern dance, yoga, and orthopedic exercise that looks deceptively easy but, believe me, is a *killer*. There's no heavy lifting and no machines; instead, light weights and the body itself are used for resistance. In my class, there are women in their fifties, sixties, and up, so it's truly an activity you can do forever. The movements are small, controlled, and intense—and, like Pilates, are great for spot-targeting problem zones. The technique is famous for what they call their "heart-shaped rear end," and for the added bonus of devotees' claims to having better sex! Maybe that's why it's so difficult to find room in a class! (See Resources.)

JOIN THE DYNA BAND BAND   Dyna-Bands are my "go-anywhere" exercise essential. They come in three color-coded thicknesses—offering varying degrees of resistance—and you can get them in any sports store. They're like giant elastic bands—but they'll never snap.

You can use Dyna-Bands for arm exercises, chest exercises, and leg exercises. The resistance they offer means they give your muscles a workout that's equivalent to lifting weights. Nobody's going to carry two five-pound weights around in her handbag but Dyna-Bands weigh almost nothing, so they're great to keep in your office drawer, your gym bag, even your handbag. This really is a double-duty exercise: you can use Dyna-Bands while you're doing other things. Put one on as you're doing the dishes. Keep them at your desk and take a few seconds out. Instead of hitting the coffee machine, do an upper body workout sitting right there—an instant energy booster without the caffeine comedown.

DYNA-BANDS FOR BREASTS

1 Hold the two ends of the Dyna Band at bust level
2 Pull your arms apart ten times. For more resistance, hold your hands closer together. Work up to three sets.

DYNA BANDS FOR ARMS

. . . are a great flab-fighter for the underarm area.

1 Hold the Dyna Band in one hand.
2 Bend your elbow and place the hand holding the Dyna Band behind your head.
3 Put your other hand in the small of your back and grab hold of the other end of the Dyna Band.
4 Straighten the top arm—feeling the resistance in the muscle that runs from the elbow to your underarm. Do a set of ten, then change hands. In all, do three sets of ten, alternating.

(A variation on a theme is to take a full water bottle in your hand and bend that arm behind your head. Then raise and lower. Repeat ten times, then switch hands.)

LEG PRESS

Lie on your back. Raise bent legs and hug them underneath your knees and into your chest. Rock gently side-to-side. Then place one leg, knee bent, on the ground. Loop a DynaBand or a towel around the ball of your other foot; pull it towards you and try to straighten the leg, keeping both hips firmly on the floor.

BICYCLING AS A METAPHOR FOR LIFE
When I lived in France, I spent my weekends in Normandy at the 150-year-old farmhouse of the French film director Claude Lelouch and his wife. Claude is a fanatical cyclist. So every weekend, we would head out on a bicycling adventure to the neighboring villages situated high up in the surrounding hilltops. Claude knew I was learning about meditation at the time and one day he said to me, "You know, you don't have to go off to India to gain a philosophy about life. You can save a lot of money, too—because all you have to do to know about life is to get on your bike." He revealed, "Bicycling is a metaphor for life."

"When biking along the flatland," he explained, "it's like the easy part of life." You don't have much pressure, you can look to the right and to the left, taking in all that you see. This is the time you are filling yourself up with pleasurable moments for the journey ahead. So take your time and enjoy yourself. But as you look ahead in the distance, you see a hill looming on the horizon. "The hill," he continued, "is like one of life's many problems; you know it's coming so you prepare yourself to attack it." You can't battle the hill (or your problem) too early, or too late. He explained, "You must hit the hill with precise timing to begin the climb in the correct spirit." I found this fascinating, as I always seemed to attack the hills we approached too early—and was then exhausted by the time I was halfway up.

The ascent of our hills was arduous and grueling. The incline was so darn tough that I was virtually biking sideways, zigzagging up the hill, gaining inches at a time. He pointed out that this is like the most difficult part of life—you gain slowly over time, inch by inch, but you never give up the pressure of moving forward. I thought I was going to die as I looked up at the last few feet. I didn't feel I had enough in me to make it to the top. Insistently, with great belief, Claude yelled encouragement. "Yes! Yes! You can do it!" The relief, the incredible sense of victory when I finally got to the top of the hill and the edge of the town, was overwhelmingly sweet. "Ahh!" he said. "And isn't that just like life? No matter how difficult you thought it was, with perseverance, you finally conquer those impossible obstacles and beat the odds."

We then rode easily through the flat terrain of the town high up in the tiny mountaintop. I was still sweaty and red-faced from my effort, but proud of my win. "Now, get ready for your reward," he twinkled. When we reached the edge of town, we were looking down the other side of the hill at the steep incline below us. I let go over the rim of the town and floated downward, gathering speed, released from all of the memories of the struggle it took to get there . . . coasting, free as a bird.

The momentum of life will take you along. So let yourself go and enjoy the ride. Know that there will be flat land where you can work on yourself and gather strength, gaining the tools and the reserve to draw on to be able to attack the many hills ahead.

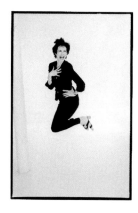
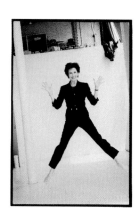
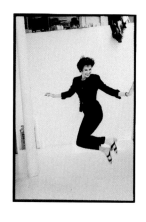
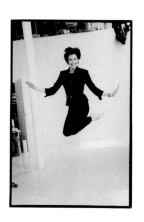

INSTANT ENERGY

These are my "quick-ups": How I rev myself up when my get-up-and-go got up and went.

- A twenty-minute walk—especially when it's the last thing I feel like doing. That's when I know it will do me the most good.
- A bottle of water. If I'm exhausted and craving coffee, I find that bottled water is the perfect pick-me-up instead. Water does the trick even if I'm not consciously thirsty. You have to keep water in sight—at your desk, on your table, by your bed. Otherwise, we forget to drink.
- An Evian water spray, spritzed on my face, instantly revives me. I carry a tiny one with me for instant pick-ups.
- In natural food stores, look for aromatherapy room mists specially designed to revive and energize. Just spray them into the air and their wonderful ingredients (like peppermint oil and eucalyptus) will do the rest! Jasmine oil is said to be the most uplifting of all the essential oils (see Heaven Scent, p.176). Put a drop on your skin and feel your energy rise.

- If I'm nervous or even a little full after a meal, I lace up my tennis shoes and jump up and down (about fifty times). Anything that oxygenates the blood and gets it circulating will give you instant energy—just enough to rev up your heartbeat and kick start your body. (It literally changes your mind.)
- My newest discovery is my mini-trampoline. It's fun, quite portable, and cost me only $49.99 (see Resources). I turn on the music, hop on, and jump a hundred times—or I'll bounce while I'm watching the news. It's great aerobic exercise, easy on the joints, and really fun!
- The salutation to the moon (see Salutation to the Moon, p.157) —or any kind of catlike stretching—gets the energy flowing again.

- One of the easiest ways to boost your energy is with light. So throw open the shades or add an extra lamp to a dark room. Let there be light!—and feel an instant lift.
- Getting into Nature, even if it's just for five minutes, has amazing results. It's good for the soul. It's also great after a big meal or before going to sleep.
- Five big inhales and exhales. We forget to breathe properly all during the day, but it re-oxygenates everything and is a bonus for the skin.
- Don't smoke. Smoking actually causes fatigue, as it depletes the amount of oxygen in your bloodstream.
- Try to find something to laugh about—there's no better medicine.

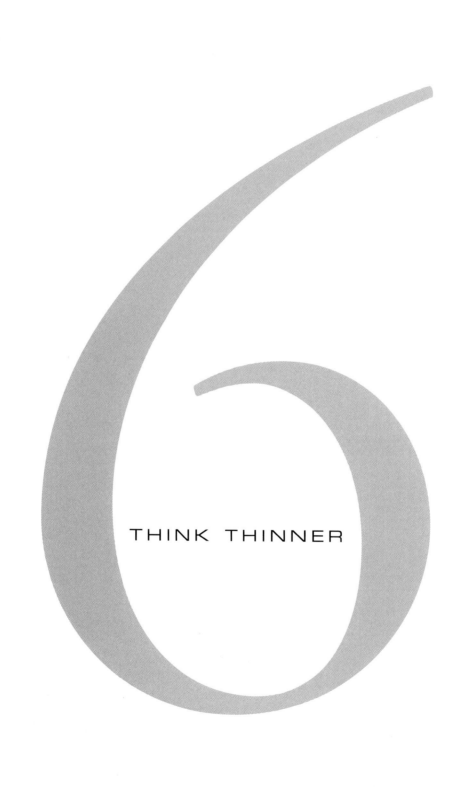

THINK THINNER

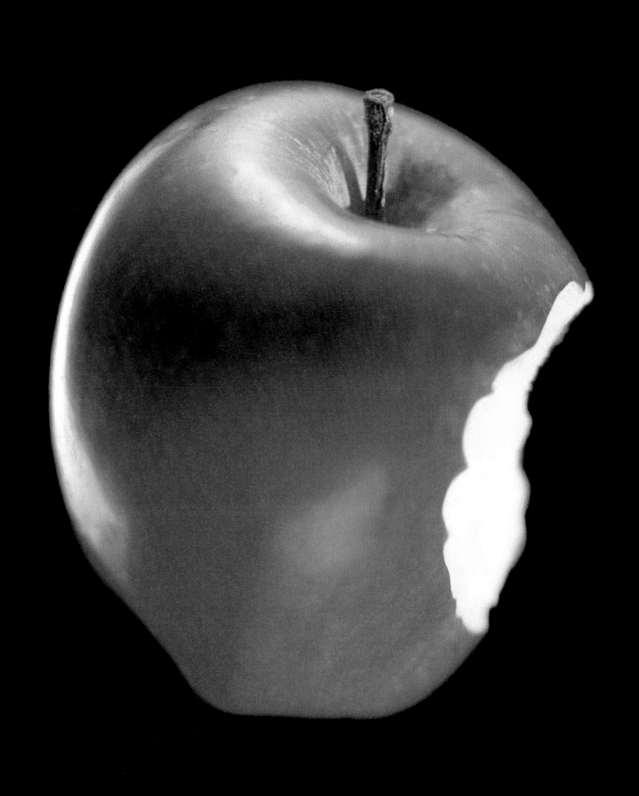

THINK
ABOUT
FOOD

IT'S ABOUT TIME . . .

. . . to throw away diets forever and discover the joy of fabulous, nutritious food. That means eating for long-term health—not to fit into a dress by Saturday. It means discovering the foods—and the vitamins—that deliver the greatest health bonus. And it certainly doesn't mean deprivation—which will send any of us scurrying for the cookie jar before long. (Guaranteed.) Over the years, I have evolved a delicious and a nutritious way of eating that keeps weight almost effortlessly at bay. It works for my friends. Believe me: It can work for you.

I've tried every diet ever invented—and broken all of them. So, over the years, I have designed my own eating "lifestyle," and it's been extremely successful, not just for me but for friends who have always failed with diets before. My good friend Michele has struggled with her weight all her life, but since she has followed my eating plan, she has gone down two dress sizes—and, *most important*, kept it off easily, she says. The secret is not dieting but thinking about proper eating as a lifestyle choice for the rest of your life. Losing weight and maintaining energy long-term means revising eating patterns forever.

The key is to learn to eat differently. Sharply restricting calories—as "diet gurus" told us to do for decades—puts the body into starvation mode. Your body panics because it doesn't know it's on a diet; it thinks it's stranded in the Sahara—and slows the rate at which it burns calories (metabolism), so that it becomes increasingly harder to lose pounds. So when you start eating normally again, you really pile on the weight, even if you're back to eating the same number of calories as before you dieted—because your body's "thermostat" is fixed at a new, lower metabolic rate.

My eating lifestyle isn't about deprivation. It's about focusing on a healthy, fun way of eating that is both satisfying and energizing; it's about food that nourishes the soul as well as the body. When I tell friends about this way of eating, I try to encourage them to think of their body as something separate from themselves, something special they are responsible for, almost like a child. That way, it's easier to start taking better care of themselves. With this heightened feeling of care, you may also listen to your body more carefully. When I'm cooking supper, ordering takeout, or dining in a restaurant, I ask my self, "What do I need to eat?" (Half the time, it's your eyes that want a cookie, not your tummy.) When you finally do get in touch with your body's needs, you'll probably find that you are drawn to eat more seasonally: strawberries in spring, salads in summer, root vegetables in winter, and apples in the fall, which is when nature intended for us to eat them. I also try to avoid foods and drinks that don't give me nutritional benefits—so-called junk food, diet products, and empty calories. You might as well be eating Styrofoam.

As we age, we must modify how we eat to avoid putting on weight and developing the classic flabbiness known as "middle-age spread." But we also have to be realistic about what our bodies should and could look like at any given age. During the menopausal years, many of us put on a layer of fat in the stomach and hip area; how hard do you want to work to keep a little softness completely at bay? Three hours of exercise a day? Four? Five? Thanks—but no

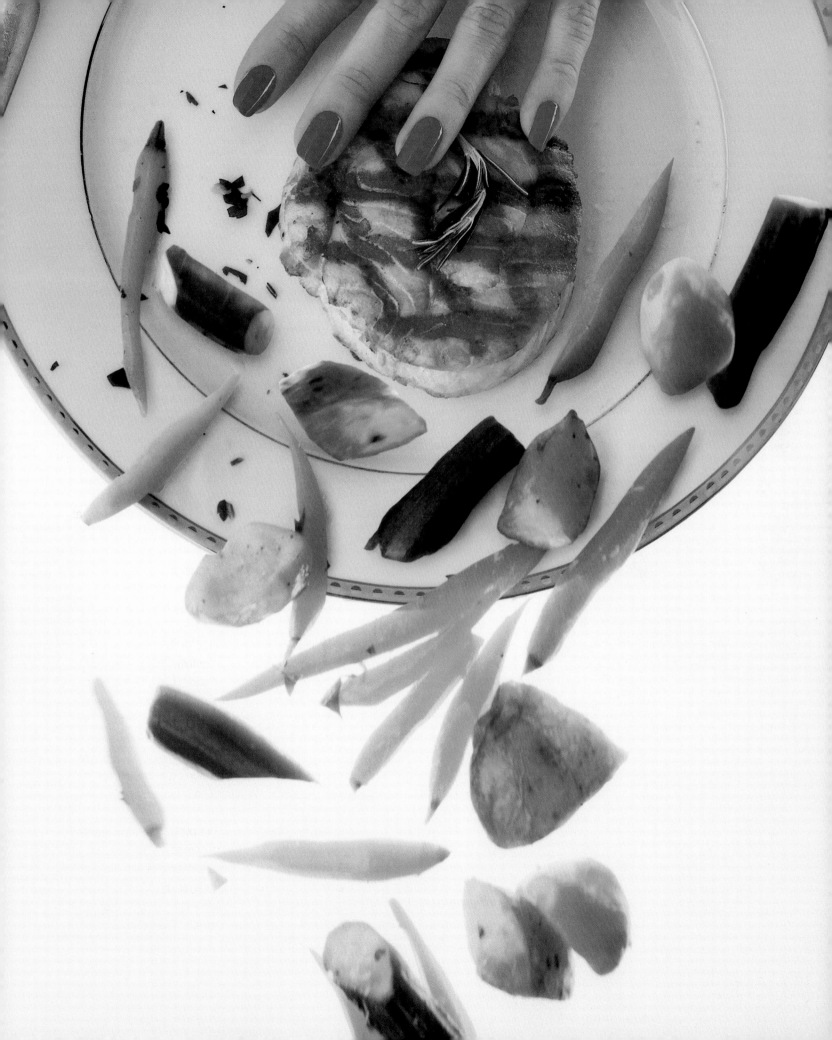

BEWARE OF THE BREAD
BOX: Personally, I find that
cutting down on bread helps
me keep weight off—not only
because I'm not getting the
calories from the extra bread,
but because I'm also avoiding
the sweet and fattening
spreads we use on them.
If you have bread, make sure
that it's as wholesome as
possible—wholegrain, preferably organic, if you can get it.
If I am going to have an occasional bagel, I will scoop out
the extra dough . . . and hold
the cream cheese. The best
toppings for breads are the
all-fruit spreads—Polaner
All-fruit and Smuckers make
delicious all-fruit spreads—
a really natural no-fat treat!

thanks. Things do change as we age. Gravity keeps tugging, lifestyles evolve, and your genes get more stubborn and harder to combat. This is all natural.

But maintaining a healthy weight is important because the emphasis is on *health*. If you eat right and maintain muscle strength, flexibility, and cardio-vascular fitness, you will add years to your life.

So, here are the guidelines for Dayle's Eating Lifestyle. The bottom line? Think long-term health, not short-term diet.

FIGHT FAT One of the biggest keys to losing weight (and keeping it off) is to cut down on fat. All calories are not created equal: The body really doesn't have to work very hard to convert the fat you eat into the fat you wear! Fat con-tains far more calories per gram than carbohydrates or protein, which serve up four calories per gram. Fat contains nine calories per gram. So cutting out fat is the fastest way to nip middle-age spread in the bud (or the butter dish).

MY TRICKS

• When I eat any kind of meat, I strip the fat off. The skin comes off the chicken, and I try to stick with white meat, which has less calories than dark meat. If I have prosciutto (which I love!) I'll take all the fat off that, too. Ground beef comes with fat content clearly marked on the labels; stick with the lower-fat sirloins. Also, blot or drain the fat off meat after you cook it.

• I don't keep butter in the house—but I do have a great butter-flavored replacement called I Can't Believe It's Not Butter Spray, available in most grocery stores. Squirt it onto your food for the taste of butter without the fat and calories. I love it on toast, vegetables, and potatoes.

• I love my little spritzer of olive oil, the Eco Pump, which I discovered at Canyon Ranch. Simply spray the oil right onto steamed vegetables. The pump limits the amount of oil that goes on so you have all the taste of olive oil with few of the calories (see Resources).

• I always use Pam spray for cooking, instead of butter or oil.

• Don't assume that food will be grilled or steamed; always ask. And be sure to request all sauces and dressings on the side; this way you can control the calories and still enjoy the flavors. A little dip often yields the same sensory expe-rience as a sea of sauce, with a fraction of the consequence. I also try to steer clear of the "aises"—Bernaise, Hollandaise, Lyonnaise, mayonnaise. To me, "aise" spells "fat."

• If my food arrives loaded with excess grease, I will dab or wipe it with a paper napkin. You'll be amazed at what you can mop up. (I even blot a ham-burger. I'm sure I absorb at least fifty calories of pure fat each time I do.)

• Beware of foods that "hide" their fat content…muffins, crackers, croissants, and cookies, to name a few. If you doubt their greasiness, just place one on a paper napkin for a few minutes and watch the oily circle that forms underneath.

SNACK ATTACK   I'm a big believer in healthy snacking during the day. One of the reasons many of us overeat or binge is because we're suffering from low blood sugar. Several hours after a meal, blood sugar can drop enough to let fatigue, or even a feeling of having the blues, set in. Often, by the time we're supposed to eat again, we're weak and ravenous, so we either wait and gorge at mealtime, or break down and pick at all the wrong foods: cookies, candy, chips, ice cream. One of the worst mistakes we make is skipping breakfast; we think we're saving calories, but we're actually setting ourselves up for day-long disasters. By eating regularly and snacking healthily between meals, we can avoid that desperate, hypoglycemic raid on the cookie jar. In fact, it's been established that the cholesterol level of nibblers is lower, which is another reason for super-snacking.

Never, ever skip a meal or deprive yourself. Think about spreading your meals out over the day. At breakfast, have a great health cereal, skim milk and orange juice—and save your banana for a morning break. Instead of eating that apple with your sandwich at lunchtime, save it for a late afternoon snack—a blood sugar equalizer (mine plummets around 4 P.M.). At suppertime, hold off on dessert—for instance, a baked apple crisp with low-fat yogurt—for a wonderful snack later in the evening.

MORE TIPS
•   If it's mealtime and you're not actively hungry, try to eat a little something healthy anyway. This helps keep that blood sugar level steady and gets you into the habit of eating regularly.
•   Try to eat your meals at more or less the same time each day. There is a lot to say about regularity at mealtime and it is much better for digestion.
•   Make your food look appetizing. Experiment with garnishes: finely chopped peppers, capers, fruit, parsley—anything that makes healthy food look more inviting. Ruby, the chef at Canyon Ranch, takes leftover pieces of brightly colored vegetables, dices them finely, and stores them in the fridge. She dips into this mixture as a final sprinkle over a finished meal before serving and, voilá! Ordinary transformed into extraordinary.
•   Add texture to food to make it more fun and interesting: sesame, sunflower, and pumpkin seeds. For breakfast, I love yogurt sprinkled with wheat germ, sunflower seeds, and fresh berries for satisfying crunch and color.
•   Toasting rice cakes makes them more tasty; a great alternative for toast.
•   It's a fact: If you've got it in the house, someday you'll eat it. But what the eye doesn't see, your tummy won't desire. My trainer, Sean, taught me this seemingly obvious, yet powerful trick: Don't buy it! There will always be that moment when you're hungry; you open the pantry door and see Oreos taunting you. Get rid of all the high-fat, high-sugar food in your house that might tempt you.
•   Always grocery shop when you're not hungry. Everything looks good when we are starving.
•   The stress-free, time-saving way to cook and eat healthy food is to prepare key ingredients for the week's meals on a Sunday. Chop fresh vegetables, includ-

CHRISTINE'S LOWER FAT BISCOTTI

When I tasted my friend Christine's biscotti (my favorite snack— I love the crunch!) I knew I had to have it in my book. Christine took a low-fat cooking class in Los Angeles and this is her favorite recipe she learned — and it's now mine (and yours)!

$1/2$ stick unsalted butter at room temperature
$2/3$ cup sugar or a bit less
2 large eggs
1 tablespoon grappa (Grand Marnier)
$1/2$ teaspoon anise extract (almond)
$11/2$ teaspoons cold water
1 to 2 teaspoons aniseed
2 cups plus 2 tablespoons flour or a bit more if dough is too soft, plus flour to roll logs
$11/2$ teaspoons baking powder
pinch salt

Preheat oven to 325°

Cream butter until fluffy, then add sugar and mix. Add eggs one at a time and combine well. Beat in grappa, extract and aniseed. Combine remaining ingredients and blend; do not overmix. Make long rolls about $11/2$ inches in diameter and place on parchment-lined cookie sheets. Bake 20 to 25 minutes or until lightly browned. Cool 5 to 10 minutes, then slice diagonally $1/2$ inch thick and bake again 10 to 15 minutes on each side or until edges feel crisp, raising temperature if not browning enough. Cool on racks.

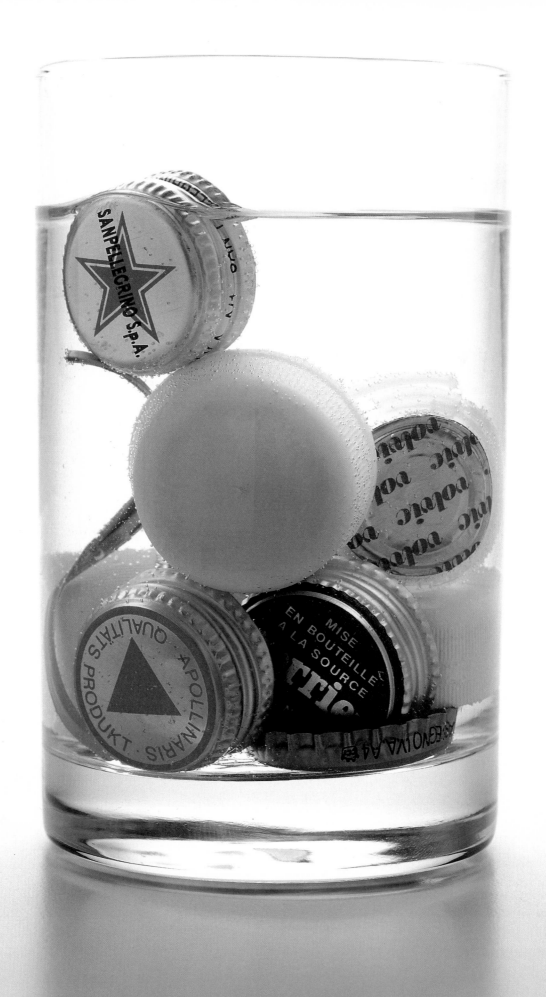

ing onions, in advance—and put them into Tupperware containers. If it's easy for you to cook fresh food during the week, you'll be less likely to order a pizza or hit the grocery store for high-fat convenience foods.

• Find ways to comfort and reward yourself other than with food. Some of my favorite treats are the Magic Bath (see p. 150), a great book, meditation, or walking in nature.

• Some women find that creative visualization helps them lose weight. This literally means imagining yourself (realistically of course) with a better body. The idea is that creative visualization removes some of the mental stumbling blocks and negative attitudes that exist between us and our goal—in this instance, a slimmer silhouette or a stronger physique. But do be realistic. At fifty or sixty, what's achievable has changed—and change isn't necessarily bad.

SWEET DREAMS   I have a sweet tooth—but I don't like artificial sweeteners; not only do I think they perpetuate addiction to sweet things, but I don't think they're healthy. Instead of regular sugar, I buy fructose (fruit sugar) from a natural food store; it gives me the sweetness I crave on cereals and in drinks, but is chemical-free and metabolized more slowly. Of course, it's possible to wean yourself off sugar altogether. But don't try to go "cold turkey"; gradually reduce the amount of sugar you take in your tea, coffee, whatever, so that your palate adjusts.

WATER, WATER   Water is one of those totally wonderful things in life. It fills you up. It helps flush out your system. It's the ultimate thirst quencher. It's natural and has zero calories. (I've been told that drinking plenty of water even helps us think more clearly, as our brains are 75 percent water and even minor dehydration can impair cognition.) What else can I say? Drink plenty of it: six to eight glasses a day. (Drink even more when traveling on a plane or to high altitudes.) Diet drinks may contain no calories, but they are full of chemicals and totally devoid of any nutritional value. When you're not drinking water, a great alternative is fresh carrot juice and freshly juiced fruits.

PROTEIN POWER   I am a protein person; if I don't get enough, I feel weak. So I try to cut my calories by reducing fats, not by skimping on protein. Although most of us eat more than enough protein, nearly 20 percent of women eat less than 30 g daily (the RDA is 50 g a day for a 140-pound woman). A study at the Gene Meyer Human Nutrition Center on Aging at Tufts University followed two groups of women: one group ate about half their RDA of protein while the others ate a little more than the RDA for protein, over the same time period. At the end of the study, the women on the low protein regimen had lost muscle, lean body weight, and actual strength—just what you don't want to lose. Their immune response was also lower.

Good sources of protein include grains, beans, cereals, seeds, eggs (I often use the whites and toss the yolk), and meat. If you do moderate weight training, it will also help you retain and use that protein better. (Lifting weights on a regular basis helps women—even older women—combat the bone-thinning effects of osteoporosis.)

BONE-SAVING FOODS

It's crucial that our diets include enough calcium, which is vital for protecting bones against the ravages of osteoporosis. To ward off this disease, the National Osteoporosis Foundation recommends 1,000 mg of calcium a day after the age of twenty-five, and 1,500 mg a day for post-menopausal women who aren't on hormone replacement therapy (HRT offers some protection against osteoporosis). Along with plenty of calcium-rich foods, you need to make sure you're taking magnesium supplements and getting enough vitamin D, which are essential for calcium absorption. (Good sources of vitamin D—shrimp, salmon, shark, swordfish, and other oily fish.)

GOOD CALCIUM SOURCES

	Milligrams of Calcium Per Serving
Milk (1 cup)	300
Calcium-fortified orange juice (1 cup)	300
Tofu (firm tofu, 1.5 oz)	300
Nonfat yogurt (1/2 cup)	225
Dried figs (5)	135
Spinach (1/2 cup, cooked)	105
Kale (1/2 cup, cooked)	89
Baked beans (1/2 cup, cooked)	80
Orange	54
Broccoli (1/2 cup, cooked)	49

At the same time, be aware that certain factors rob our bodies of vital calcium supplies or affect the way we absorb this essential mineral:

- A diet that's high in fat, sodium, or protein
- Caffeine and cola drinks
- Cigarette smoking
- Inadequate acid in the stomach for digestion (a doctor can test for this)
- An excess of fiber from grains and bran
- Certain drugs and over-the-counter medications

HITTING YOUR HEALTHY WEIGHT . . . AND STAYING THERE

The good news is that today most doctors are being a little more generous when it comes to determining what our healthy weight should be. But I strongly believe that we have to make a shift away from seeing weight in terms of poundage and from making ourselves crazy over day-to-day fluctuations. So throw out those scales (or at least stow them in the closet). For instance, if you're starting to exercise, you may lose inches as you strengthen your body, but the scales may reveal a misleading signal since muscle weighs more than fat. How demoralizing is that? Focus on how good you feel in your clothes after you

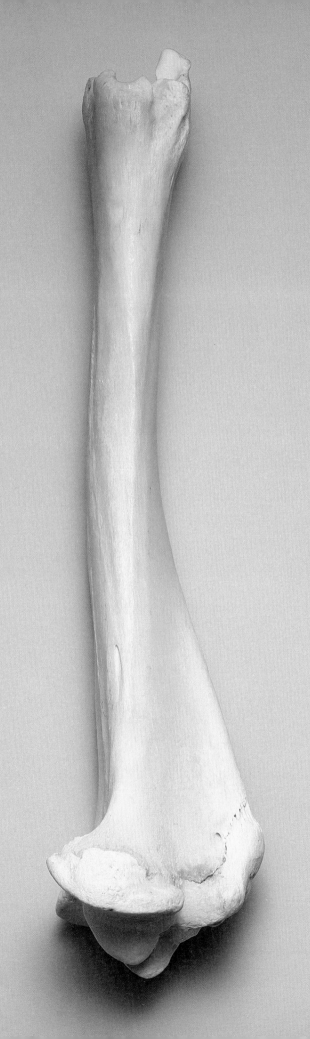

have worked out instead of measuring progress by the number that comes up on a scale. None of us, when we look in the mirror, sees the truth, but there's no escaping how comfortable (or miserable!) we can feel in our favorite pair of jeans.

I don't believe in setting radical weight-loss goals, either. It's like saying, "I'm going to climb Mount Kilimanjaro." It is impossible to imagine how you're going to get up there from here. So many studies have shown that if you lose weight quickly, you'll put it right back on. So the key is to do it gradually, one step at a time, which is just how you'd climb Kilimanjaro. Psychologically, it's no longer deprivation, but a positive move. It becomes a way of life, not another regimen.

This is the time in life to develop a realistic approach to food—seeing it as the ally in the war against aging, not as the enemy (which is how many women still regard food). At this stage, we should be getting in touch with our bodies, managing our diets to maximize the perfect fuel foods and drinks, and be aware of how food makes us feel after we eat.

SUPERSNACKS

Organize your refrigerator and your cupboard so that you have healthy snacks on hand when the munchies strike. Go for tasty, high-fiber foods that are low in fat and sugar:

- Chopped fruit.
- A few small crackers with a little bit of All American Spoon Fruit (fruit spread) or low-fat peanut butter skimmed across it.
- Roasted soya beans (from natural food stores). I keep these in my bag and if I'm hungry rushing around during the day, I grab a handful.
- Cut up carrots, celery, cauliflower, mushrooms, broccoli, or peppers. Store them in handy Ziploc baggies—alternating so you don't get bored. Anyone who's rejected vegetable snacks should try again with organic produce. Organic vegetables are much tastier and therefore far more satisfying.
- Balance Bars (a nutritional food bar)—another of my favorites. In a pinch, they are a great source of energy and nutrition, so I like to keep one in my purse at all times! They're a great boost before a workout, too. I love the chocolate and honey peanut flavors (see Resources).
- If you absolutely have to have french fries, try them the Oprah way: Brush the sliced potatoes with a little egg white for crispness and bake in the oven for 40 to 45 minutes.
- Instant oatmeal is more than a snack, it's a mini-meal. Sprinkle the oatmeal with raisins or seeds. Be creative.
- Popcorn—air popped without fat, then sprinkled with (a little) salt. (My friend Colleen takes hers with her to the movies!)
- Wax Orchards' OH Fudge chocolate sauce really satisfies chocolate cravings, but is actually made from grapes. It is wonderful warmed up and spooned over Columbo frozen yogurt, which is how they serve it at Canyon Ranch: ninety calories for two tablespoons (see Resources).

CHOPPED FRUIT
CRACKERS
SOYA BEANS
VEGETABLES
FUDGE
FRENCH FRIES
OATMEAL
POPCORN
BALANCE BARS

VITAMINS

Vitamin A

or beta-carotene   4000 IU

Vitamin C   60 mg

(Personally, I take 1,000 mg daily)

Vitamin E   10 IU

Vitamin D   400 IU

Vitamin B1

or thiamin   1.5 mg

Vitamin B2

or riboflavin   1.7 mg

Niacin   19 mg

Vitamin B6

or pyridoxine   2.0 mg

Folic acid   200 mcg

Vitamin B12   2.0 mcg

Pantothenic acid   4–7 mg

Biotin   30–100 mcg

MINERALS

Iron   0–15 mg

Calcium   800–1200mg

Phosphorus   1200 mg

Manganese   .50–2.0 mg

Iodine   150 mcg

Copper   1.5–3.0 mg

Zinc   15 mg

Chromium   50–200 mg

Selenium   70 mcg

Molybdenum   50–750 mcg

Boron   1.5–3.0 mg

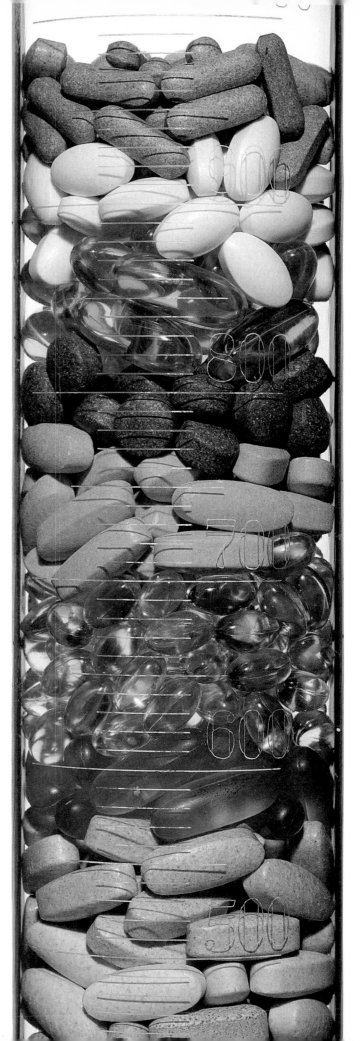

VITAL VITAMINS

Nobody has a perfect diet (even if they follow this book!). Pollution, cigarette smoking, stress, and the aging process itself can cause vitamin and mineral deficiencies.

In an ideal world, we'd get all we need from our food. This is not an ideal world. Nevertheless, I still try to get as many of my vitamins as possible from my food by keeping my diet truly varied. I like to keep up to date with the latest nutritional thinking through the *Harvard Medical Review* and the MAYO Clinic newsletter, among others. If you can, read up on vitamins in magazines, newspapers, journals; try things for yourself and feel (and see, in the mirror) whether they make a difference. I will listen to a recommendation from a friend I trust and try it out. If you're unsure about what you should and shouldn't be taking, particularly if you're on medication from your doctor, consult with her or find a naturopath who can advise you. (Natural food stores are usually up-to-date about your local alternative practitioners who may be worth seeing.)

WHAT'S A FREE RADICAL? You will often hear free radicals and aging mentioned in the same breath. They are molecules with one missing electron. They are the enemy: "cellular terrorists" that attack healthy cells in order to replace the missing electron and complete themselves. Free radicals are created by all the things we want to avoid: stress, pollution, smoking, and UV exposure. Many health care professionals (and skin-care companies like L'Oréal) are now convinced that free radicals contribute to skin aging. But here's the good news: Nature has equipped us to fight free radicals with antioxidants, which is why skin creams are increasingly being formulated to incorporate antioxidant vitamins. So we can fight the anti-aging war two ways: externally and internally. The creams tackle the surface damage, and antioxidant vitamins, particularly beta-carotene, C, E, and selenium, taken orally, help undo some of the harm that free radicals wreak internally, which is vital, since not only are they linked with wrinkles, but with heart disease, some kinds of arthritis, and maybe cancer, too.

THE BASICS If you want to get the most of your vitamins and minerals in one easy-to-take pill, look for one that provides at least 10 to 12 minerals and 11 to 12 vitamins at doses of 100 to 200 percent of the Recommended Daily Allowance (RDA). Scan the labels of supplements and compare them to the chart. These are the basics that will maintain a good level of nutrition insurance, even if you're stressed.

TIP

At the very least, almost everyone could do with a multi-vitamin/multi-mineral supplement each day. My experience is that when it comes to supplements, you usually have to pay for quality: Some formulas are more easily assimilated by the body.

THE KEY ANTI-AGING SUPPLEMENTS

VITAMIN C

According to the late Dr. Linus Pauling (who lived to ninety-three!), we could all add an extra twelve to eighteen years to our lives by taking between 3,200 to 12,000 mg of vitamin C a day. Government data on the diets of 11,000 Americans showed that as much as 300 mg of vitamin C (half in supplements) added two years to a woman's life. Find C in citrus fruits, Brussel sprouts, broccoli, strawberries, and tomatoes.

ZINC

A great immune booster; if you take a zinc supplement when you feel a cold or the flu coming on, it can sometimes stop it in its tracks. (I am an avid fan of zinc lozenges for a sore throat.) It also works as an antioxidant. Food sources include shellfish, cereals, nuts, and seeds, but our ability to absorb zinc decreases with age and some zinc-rich foods contain other elements that actually reduce zinc absorption, so you may want to supplement. (Fifteen to 30 mg a day for adults is usually enough to correct deficiencies and get the immune system back on track.)

BETA-CAROTENE

Our body transforms beta-carotene into vitamin A, an immune-boosting vitamin in its own right. More than one hundred studies indicate that people with high levels of beta-carotene in their diet are roughly half as likely to develop a wide range of cancers, especially of the lung, but including throat, mouth, esophagus, breast, and bladder. Beta-carotene is also good for stroke prevention and helps slow down eye degeneration. (Carrots, it seems, really do help you to see in the dark.) Let your eyes steer you to good sources of beta-carotene; they're often bright yellow or bright red: apricots, carrots, sweet potatoes, cantaloupes, peppers. Other sources include endive, spinach, cabbage, and kale. As a rule of thumb, the darker the color, the higher the beta-carotene content.

SELENIUM

Selenium is coming up fast in the anti-aging stakes. It works as an antioxidant, and we can use all the antioxidants we can get! A deficiency in selenium is linked with an increased risk of cancer and heart disease. Selenium is also said to alleviate menopausal hot flashes. Good sources to boost your intake of selenium are grains, swordfish, tuna, oysters, Brazil nuts, garlic, and sunflower seeds..

VITAMIN E

According to varying studies, vitamin E lowers the risk of colon and other cancers, boosts immunity, fights the free radical chain reaction that destroys cells (including in our skin), and helps prevent artery clogging. In a study of 87,000 nurses, incidence of heart disease was 41 percent lower among the women who took between 100 to 125 IUs of vitamin E daily for more than two years. Food sources of vitamin E include wheat germ, whole grains, sunflower seeds, nuts, and lobster.

CALCIUM

As mentioned earlier in the osteoporosis section, calcium is a big must for the baby boomer woman. Along with iron, calcium is the mineral most deficient in the American woman's diet. What's more, for women, calcium absorption is reduced as we age—one of the factors leading to osteoporosis. Caffeine, fizzy soft colas, and cigarettes also rob the body of calcium. Ideally, calcium should be taken with magnesium; women with osteoporosis also often lack magnesium. Aim for a product with 800 mg of calcium to 400 mg of magnesium, as the two work together. Because it's often hard for the body to access the calcium in supplements, try to take them with meals or at bedtime, spreading your intake throughout the day to minimize the chances of the minerals being lost through body wastes. Good dietary sources of calcium include milk, cheese, broccoli, pulses (i.e., lentils and beans), leafy green vegetables, nuts, and seeds. *NOTE: The basic requirements for both calcium and magnesium are so high that putting them into a multisupplement would make for a real "horse pill": You almost certainly need a calcium supplement on top of a multi.*

ANTI-AGING MIRACLES

DHEA One of the real anti-aging buzz supplements, DHEA (short for dehy-droepiandrosterone) is a hormone that is believed to help combat many age-relat-ed problems: cancer, heart disease, Alzheimer's, diabetes, and a gradual running down of the immune system. DHEA levels start to drop by age twenty-five, and by sixty-five, they're only 10 to 20 percent of what they were when we were twenty. Some evidence indicates that DHEA supplementation may improve brain function, help combat memory loss, boost immunity, ease muscle fatigue and bone fragility, and perhaps up our natural protection against cancer. It's also thought to help weight loss, fighting the body's tendency to pile on pounds as we age. You will need to boost your intake of antioxidants during any DHEA therapy to minimize the risk of possible free radical damage by taking the hormone. So far as DHEA's potential as an anti-aging miracle worker is concerned, then, it's a case of watch this space.

MELATONIN The sleepless (and international travelers) may already be familiar with melatonin. It's another hormone—one which helps reset the body clock and acts like a "natural" sleeping pill, without the negative side effects of prescription drugs. After forty, the level of our body's melatonin production slows down. Because melatonin works on the pineal gland, which is like a "Mission Control" for the body's other systems, the reduction in melatonin production in our forties tells other systems to slow down, as well, whereupon aging kicks in. Various studies, however, have indicated that melatonin supplementation may be effective in helping to prevent heart disease (by reducing blood cholesterol) and could help treat (or prevent) asthma, cataracts, diabetes, and Parkinson's dis-ease. Melatonin is also a potent antioxidant, helping to prevent damage by free radicals.

GINKGO BILOBA This herb improves blood circulation and, accord-ing to many studies, boosts brain function. In older people, in particular, gingko seems to increase blood flow to the brain, improving short-term memory. (I always say that after forty, to have a great memory, you need ginkgo biloba—and a *young* assistant!)

VITAMIN Q (a.k.a. Coenzyme Q-10 or coQ-10): By the time we hit middle age, our production of this antioxidant has really dwindled. (It already starts to go into free fall at twenty.) CoQ-10 is thought to work like vitamin E, helping to fight cell damage by free radicals. Various studies have indicated that coQ-10 may lower blood pressure, boost immune functioning, and protect the brain against degenerative diseases. (Oily fish is a rich food source of coQ-10, which may explain why fish is considered to be a heart- and brain-boosting food.) It's considered extremely safe to take, with no side effects—but of course, if you're on medication, you should talk to your doctor. (An added bonus of taking coQ-10 is that it helps heal gum disease, which is more common as we age.)

I find that an occasional dose of ginseng acts as a wonderful tonic and energizer. The most easily absorbed forms of ginseng are liquid extracts or capsules, but you can chew a thin slice of dried root, three times a day; you can find these in natural food stores. GINSENG has a reputation as a rejuvenating tonic and a longevity herb that delays the aging process—partly because ginseng, too, is an antioxidant. It's especially useful during menopause when stress is contributing to symptoms such as hot flashes. But be warned: Avoid caffeine and other stimulants when taking ginseng and only take it for short periods—no more than two to three months at a time. Many practioners believe that DONG QUAI—a.k.a. dang gui—is a much better tonic herb for women than ginseng, which is more of a "masculine" herb (ginseng is actually known as "man herb"). Like ginseng, Dong quai is particularly useful in menopause; it also works to aid circulation, speed tissue repair, lower blood pressure, slow the pulse, help prevent atherosclerosis and blood clots—and relax the muscles of the heart. What's more, it helps the absorption of vitamin E. So it's useful to take these together.

When I'm feeling a little low or run down, I don't run to the doctor until I've tried some of these alternatives:

- EmergenC-Lite (from natural food stores) is a packet of vitamins and trace minerals that gives instant uplift. (It's also terrific if you happen to have had one glass too many the night before.)
- If I'm traveling abroad, sometimes I take supplements that help the digestive system to stay healthy—acidophilus and bifidus—from natural food stores. When I traveled to India for three months, I took both of these—and didn't get sick for one day. (In India, this ranks as a minor miracle.)
- If I've been to the dentist or bruised myself, I take homeopathic arnica, which is also good for shock. I also take homeopathic belladonna for a throbbing headache.
- For any kind of shock, nerves before public speaking, and other major stresses, I take Dr. Bach's Remedies Rescue Remedy (found in most vitamin or health food stores), which lives up to its name: A few drops of flower essences (distilled in alcohol) on the tongue really calms you down immediately.
- During the cold and flu season, I take echinacea (pronounced EK-IN-AY-SHA)—a Native American herbal immune-booster—or Oscillococcinum (pronounced AH-SILL-O-COX-SEE-NUM), originally from France. It's been popular there for over four years, but is now available in most pharmacies in the United States as well.
- The caffeine contained in both green and black tea is less aggressive than that in coffee, and scientists believe that certain teas may have healing benefits, too. Long used in the East as a digestion aid, green tea now is thought to help prevent a number of cancers (including stomach, esophagal, skin, lung, colon, liver, pancreas, and breast) and also contains powerful antioxidants. And according to the American Health Foundation, research is now showing that black tea may offer similar anti-aging safeguards. (Another reason to put the kettle on is that having a cup of green tea is thought to reduce the risk of heart disease and stroke, as well as cancer.)

For more information on homeopathy, see suggested reading list.

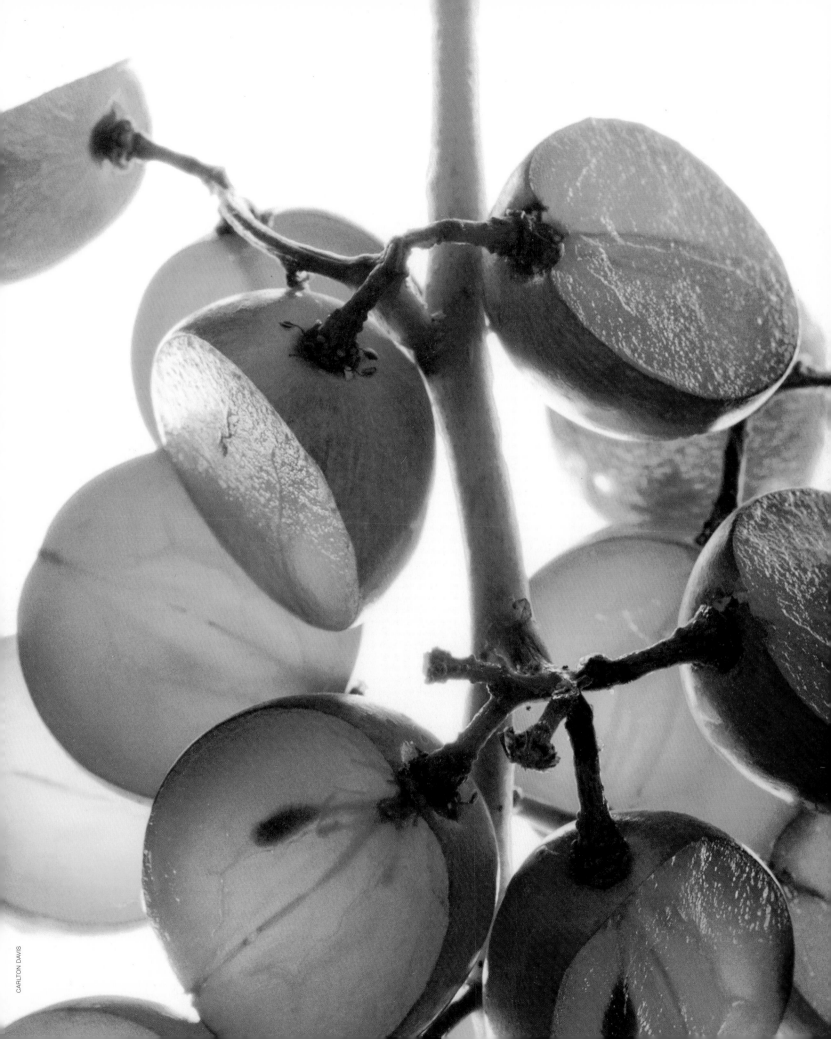

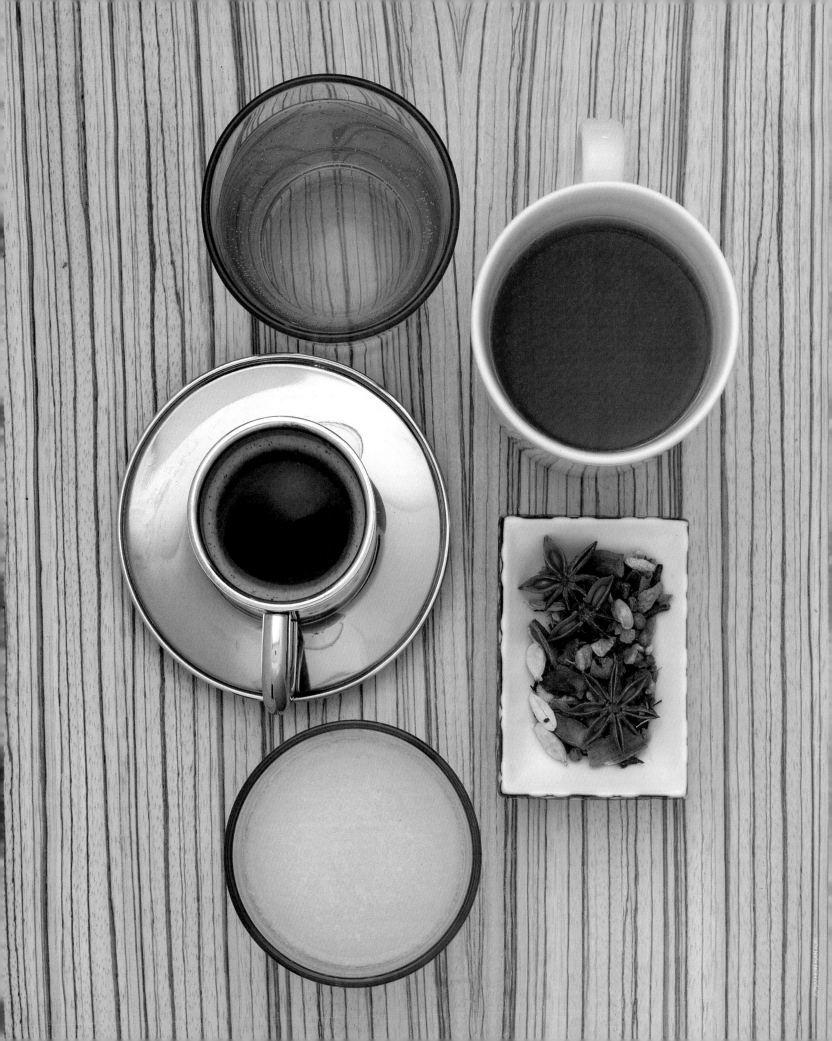

THE VICE SQUAD

Next to chocolate, my vice is coffee. I love coffee in all forms: cappuccino, latte, iced, hot, cold, espresso, and coffee yogurt. But caffeine is not great news for the body, so I try to get the pleasure of an occasional coffee without the roller-coaster mood swings. I love the highs but I hate the lows of coffee drinking. Caffeine can also hurt my stomach and make me feel jangled. I've understood for a long time that coffee is wrong for me; it interferes with the absorption of vitamins, it acts as a diuretic, and it keeps me up at night.

In the past, whenever I tried to give up coffee, I would get crushing headaches that no aspirin would relieve. (Anything that triggers that dramatic a withdrawal has to be bad for you.) But when I was visiting England a few years ago, I discovered Whole Earth Wake Cup, a grain-based coffee with guarana, which gives a more mellow and sustained lift (see Resources). I drink a cup in the morning and it picks me up right away without the jitters. And, because it is grain-based, it's nutritious, too. (They also make a version without guarana, called NoCaf, which is great late at night.) With Wake Cup, I can have an occasional cup of coffee, without being dependent on it. I'm much less tired; in the old days, by 4 P.M. I'd have to grab another cup of coffee or I couldn't finish my work.

There are many other delicious alternatives to that java jolt:

- HERBAL TEAS: Celestial Seasonings, which you can get in just about any grocery store, makes delicious herbal teas; I love the almond flavor (try it at night with milk and fruit sugar) and Roastaroma, which is actually a pretty good coffee substitute. You can make iced herbal teas in the summer and keep a pitcher of it in the fridge. I also like Japanese caffeine-free Kukicha tea and a spicy Indian tea called chai. If you keep a selection handy, you can pick and choose the perfect tea to match your mood.
- CALI TEA: This Chinese tea, made by Sunrider (see Resources), offers your body a gentle detox and, according to the company, caffeine-free energy. I like to sweeten my tea with Stivia, a natural sweetener made from chrysanthemum flower extract (also made by Sunrider).
- JUICES: I believe fresh-squeezed juices really help your skin. You can find juice bars at many health food stores, or invest in a juicer and experiment with interesting combinations: apple and carrot or celery and beet are delicious. (If you can bear wheat grass juice, which tastes like liquidized lawn clippings, only worse, it is the Rolls-Royce of juices in terms of nutritional punch.) See suggested reading list for some great books on the subject. In summer, try making homemade lemonade with fresh squeezed lemons and fruit sugar and keep a pitcher in the fridge.
- WATER: There is nothing more energizing and refreshing than water, yet we don't drink nearly enough of it. One of my favorite bottled waters is Badoit, which is just a little carbonated. I also like Vittel, Evian, and Poland Spring. After a while, it's possible to tell the difference between the brands—almost like drinking wines! If you don't want to buy bottled water, invest in a Brita water filter, available in most department stores. It's a great health investment, eliminating some of the impurities and chemicals in tap water. We are, after all, 70 percent water, and the water that flushes through the system should be as pure as possible. *NOTE: Think about making clean water ice cubes, too.*

PART TWO

BEAUTY FROM WITHIN

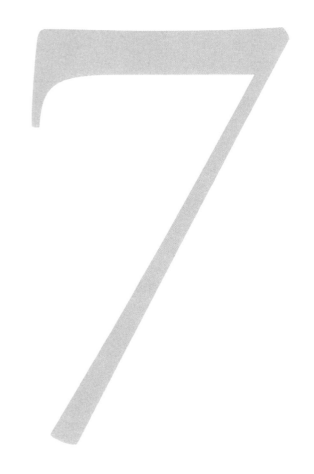

STRESS BUSTING

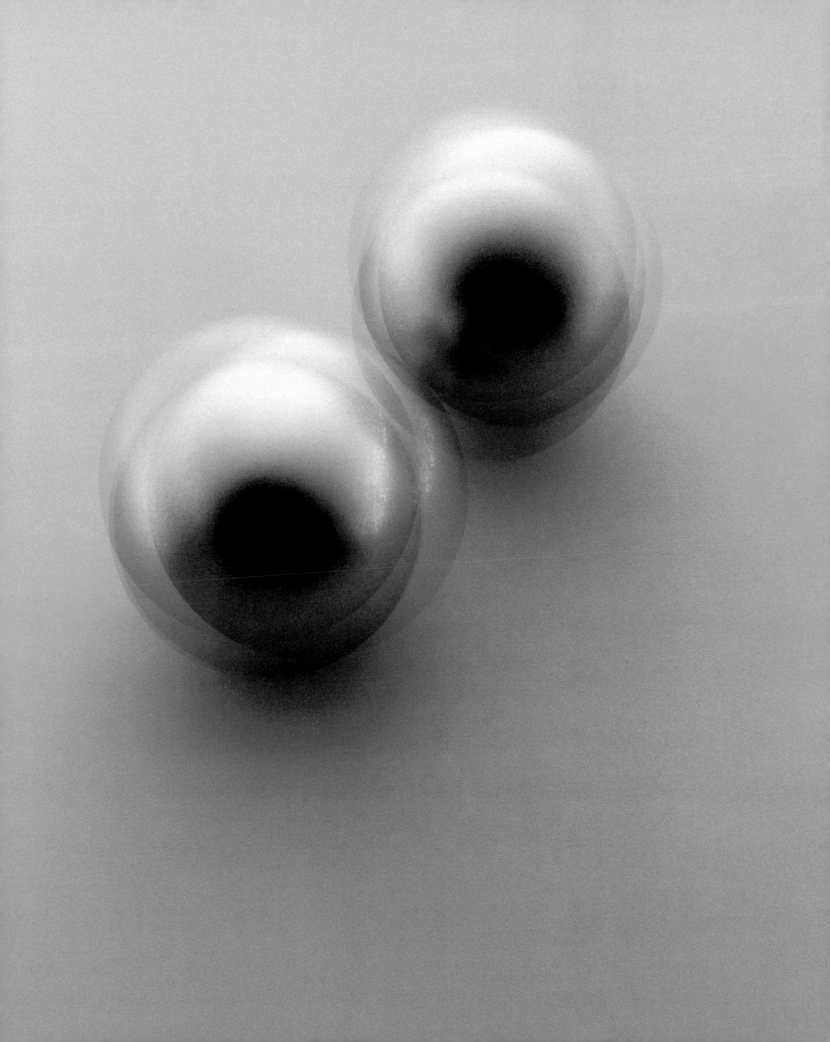

BREATHE, WOMAN

When my girlfriends come to me in a state of panic, the first thing I say is, "Breathe, woman!" You can't achieve anything in a stressed-out situation, and breathing correctly is the fastest way to calm yourself: deliberate, conscious breathing, or an exercise that incorporates breathing, like yoga. To my mind, oxygen beats Valium any day.

Breathing is something we tend to take for granted, and something we don't do well, as a rule. Not breathing properly quickly leads to exhaustion; you're not oxygenating your muscles, your organs, or your skin, and it shows. When you're anxious, you are only using the upper lungs. The air in your lower lungs is stale and probably full of toxins.

I love fresh air. In winter, I leave the windows open and pile on the covers. I fill my house with plants, which convert CO_2 into oxygen. Oxygen is good for the skin, body, and sense of well-being. (It makes me laugh that some skin creams and facials today boast of being able to deliver pure oxygen to the skin. I always thought that's what your lungs, heart, and blood are supposed to do.) It's good to get out into nature where the air is freshest—especially around trees. When I walk in the city streets and the cars and trucks belch out carbon monoxide, I will often cover my face with a scarf or my sleeve so that I don't breathe it in. (This helps to protect my skin from the aging effect of pollution, too.)

One of my fast, energy-boosting "quick-ups" is to stop what I'm doing for a moment and take three or four big, deep breaths through my nose, concentrating on pushing the air into my lower lungs. Yogic breathing is perfect for this. Most of the time, we breathe from our chests. In yoga, you learn to breathe from your diaphragm, the large, dome-shaped muscle that arches across the base of the lungs.

To learn diaphram breathing:
- Stand up straight with your feet together, shoulders down, and your hands resting on your hips.
- Inhale deeply, feeling the air push your stomach out from the diaphragm. You can literally place your hand on your stomach, just at your navel and feel it inflate like a balloon.
- Put your hands on your rib cage, feeling your ribs expand and contract like a pair of bellows as you take each breath.
- Hold, then exhale slowly. Repeat.

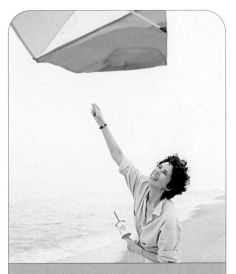

IT'S ABOUT TIME . . .

. . . to combat stress. When we move beyond stress, we can begin to get more out of life. Sure, these are stressful times. We can't always control life's angsts—but we can control how we respond to them. Since doctors estimate that 60 to 90 percent of all medical conditions are stress-related, conquering it is vital to our health, well-being, and good looks. (Frowns are not gorgeous.) Here's what works for me—and what I've taught women I know. So take a deep breath.

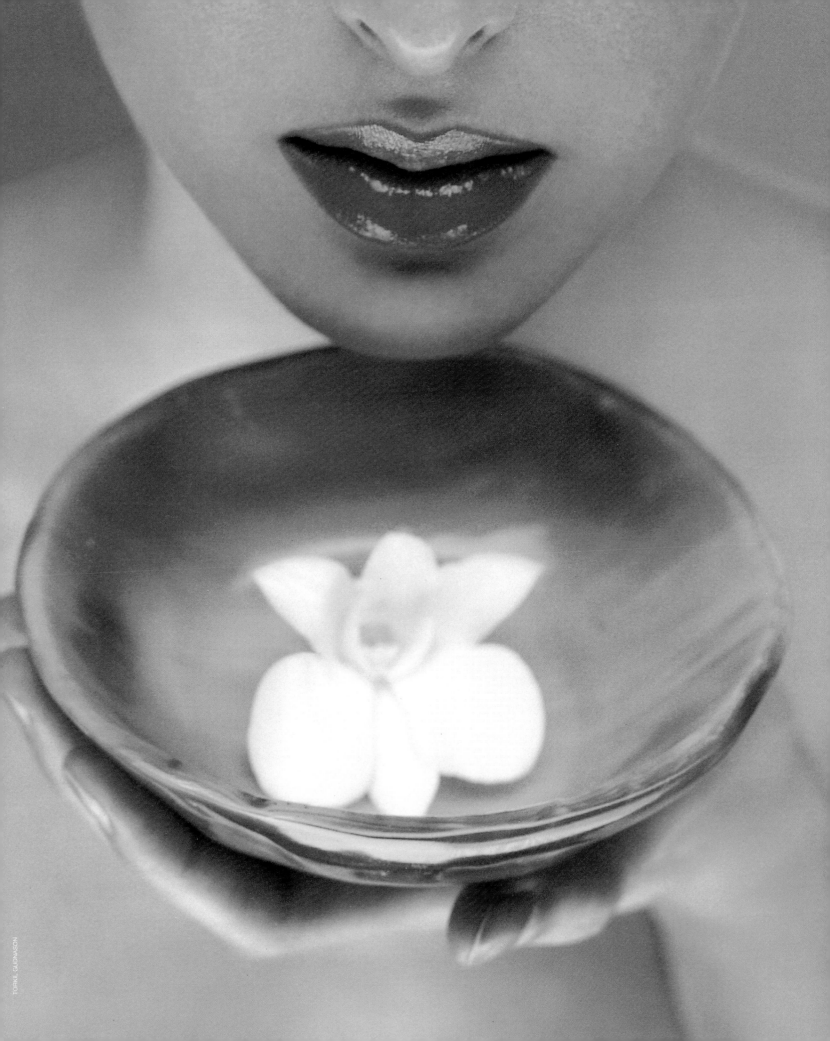

CLEAR THE AIR If you're worried about indoor air quality, especially if you live or work in a building with little fresh air, think about investing in a plug-in ionizer. It's now believed that "positive ions" (positively charged molecules) in the air can cause headaches, feelings of weakness, and worsen the condition of bronchitis or asthma. By contrast, it's thought that negative ions can "charge" a person with new vitality and energy. Electrical ionizers work on the principle that negative ions not only have a "tonic effect" on the nervous system, but also clear the air of dust particles, smoke, pollen, and smells. There is evidence to suggest that ionizers—cheap to buy and cheap to run—will provide fresher and cleaner air for you, your family, and your co-workers to breathe indoors. And if you have any doubts, just look at the dirt on the filter of a typical ionizer after only a few days of use.

Another great air improver is a humidifier. Not only will your skin love you for it, but the added moisture helps you conquer fatigue. As mentioned in Moisture Power (p. 28), I suggest buying one that holds a daily supply that you must change regularly, otherwise the machine can become a breeding ground for bacteria. Ideally, it's best to have a humidifier at home and in the office. (My recommended brand is Bionaire—see Resources.)

THE MAGIC BATH

Women often ask me how, while trying to balance busy lives, to realistically find time for self-renewal. I tell them that a fifteen-minute bath is one of my most important beauty secrets. (If fifteen minutes seems impossible, try five: It still makes a difference.) The bathroom is one place where we can close the door on the world and experience "private time." When I lived in Europe, bathing was much more a part of life than it is here, where we shower—like everything else— for speed. Some of my European friends even read their daily paper while luxuriating in a morning bath. They start their day relaxed, refreshed, *and* informed!

I hear over and over from women that they don't have time for what I believe is the infinitely rewarding indulgence of a bath. Certainly, we don't have time for everything, but I believe this should come pretty high up on the list of so-called "treats," which actually will help you re-balance your life and renew your spirit. You have to pick the things that make sense to *you*; you don't have to do them all at once, but pick one or two from time to time. There is a high return on taking a bath: It's healing, it's revitalizing—and it's fun.

If you have children, wait until they're either at school or in bed asleep. If you're single, working hard and exhausted, it may be more a case of finding the self-discipline rather than giving up and flopping in front of the TV. If you have dogs, put them in another room—they've been known to jump right in. Turn off the phone and give yourself a whole quarter of an hour! The dividend on your time investment is huge. You will feel you are valuable again. So I would say, fight for it—fight for that time and make it special. After the most hellish of days, I find I can wind down or rev up, and completely turn my day around by taking what I call my "magic bath": a ritual that includes bubbles, bath oil, candlelight, music—and sometimes a glass of wine. For most of us, showering is the fast and easy option, but even a few minutes in a bath can put a new spin on your life. I can almost watch my problems swirl down the drain.

STEP-BY-STEP TO THE MAGIC BATH   The goal of a bath is key: Do you want it to be a get-up-and-go bath or are you trying to relax and combat high stress? Would you like to reflect on and prepare for an important day ahead, speed deep sleep, or be ready for a hot night on the town? With your goal firmly in mind, draw your bath.

1   Concoct your own bath potion depending on exactly what you are feeling at the time. Aromatherapists—people who work with fragrant oils distilled from plants—say that the nose can lead you instinctively toward what your mind and body need: Sniff the bath products that you have and whichever smells best to you is what you should be using at this time. You can throw in bath salts—sometimes lavender-scented (I love Aphrodisia Naturals). You can find great bath salts in department stores, specialty bath shops, and natural food stores. Common Epsom salts is a time-tested recipe for relieving aching muscles; you can also find mineral-rich Dead Sea salts in most drugstores. Adding a tablespoon of oil—massage oil, almond oil, jojoba oil—can help fight dryness of the skin. Sprinkling in seaweed powder (again, from the bath department of department stores or natural food stores) has a detoxifying and relaxing effect and is like bringing the sea into your bathroom. Bubbles spell luxury—and the playfulness of being a child again. Part of the fun is creatively selecting and mixing *all* the ingredients so that no two baths are ever alike.

2   Next, make a selection from some of your favorite musical pieces: I like Mozart's Piano Concerto No. 21, Albinoni's Adagio, or John Coltrane to rev me up. Keep a few CDs and an inexpensive battery-operated CD player in the bathroom.

3   On stay-at-home nights, light perfumed candles or pour yourself a chilled glass of wine or sparkling mineral water and lower the lights. To make it even more comfortable, put a bath pillow (from The Body Shop) at the end of the tub for your neck; a small, rolled-up towel works just as well.

4   Keep your "goal" in mind when adjusting the bath temperature: a little hotter if you just want to let go and unwind, a little cooler in summer or anytime you're aiming for refreshment and energy.

5   Spend the first five minutes purely relaxing. Then go to work with a body brush. Starting from the toes, "polish" the skin on the body in a gentle, circular motion (see Body Brushing, p. 88). This whisks away dead cells, leaving skin soft and smooth to the touch. Polishing also boosts circulation. Be careful if you have sensitive skin, though, as the heat of the water, combined with the pressure of the brush, can cause tiny capillary vessels to break. As

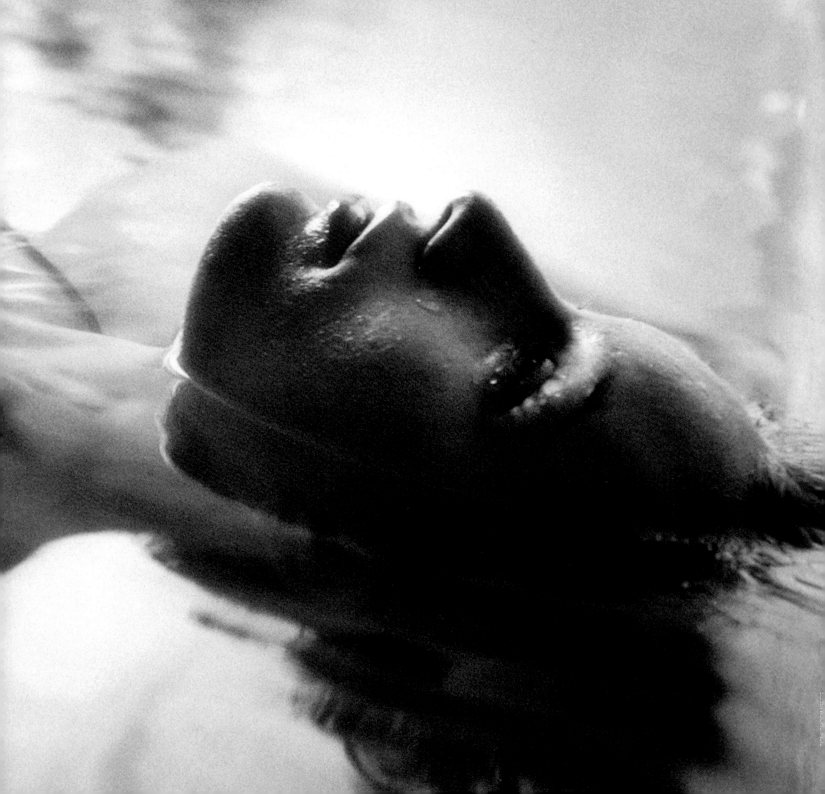

"IT IS THE SIMPLE THINGS IN LIFE
THAT ARE THE MOST EXTRAORDINARY"

PAULO COELHO

BATH
FOUGERE
SOAP

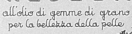
Aromathology
Relaxation
ESSENTIAL OIL BLEND
5ml e

EO™
ESSENTIAL OIL PRODUCTS
JASMINE
jasminum grandiflorum

Poudre
Dermophile
Stérilisée
DE
T. Leclerc
PARIS

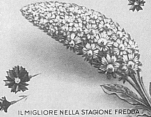
Sapone
RESEDA
all'olio di gemme di grano
per la bellezza della pelle

IL MIGLIORE NELLA STAGIONE FREDDA

VALOBRA®

BANHO
CITRON VERBENA BATH FOAM
CLAUS
PORTO

an alternative to the body brush or loofah, take a small handful of a body exfoliant (natural oatmeal or coarse kosher salt are good for sensitive and dry skin), and do the same thing.

6   Next, take a pumice stone—a lump of volcanic lava you can find at any drugstore—and scrub the really dry areas: heels, soles of your feet, and (more gently) your elbows and knees. This is also a good time to shave your legs, if that's what you do; the hairs have been softened by the water and your skin is moist, making it easier for the razor to glide over the skin without any nicks or cuts.

7   Stand up and polish the parts of your body you can't reach sitting down. It's best to start from the bottom and work toward your chest, in the direction of the heart.

8   Bathtime is a wonderful time for stretching because your muscles are already warm. Pull each knee to the chest. Lift one leg, and—with the knee to the side—gently pull that ankle toward you. (This is a wonderful stretch for the hips.) With legs straight ahead and feet flexed, try to touch your toes. Stretching in the bath, you will probably find you can reach farther than usual.

9   Rinse your skin with a little cooler water, wrap yourself in a large, fluffy bath towel or terry robe, and pat dry.

10 Your "new body" is perfectly primed for moisturizer. Give extra attention to those trouble spots: knees, elbows, feet, and hands. Massage from your toes to your neck, working in the cream until it's completely absorbed.

Now you are truly ready to hit the town—or your pillow.

ZZZZZZ . . .

At the turn of the century, people averaged nine hours of sleep a night. Now we live on seven, so it's no wonder there's a fatigue epidemic out there. When you don't get enough sleep, it's hard to do anything. I envy those people who say they can get by on five hours a night, because I think of all the things I could do with a couple of extra hours a day. But to me, eight hours (if I can manage it) is essential. While we sleep, energy levels are restored, growth, thyroid, and sex hormones surge, and the skin's rate of cell renewal is at its highest. It's also the time that the mind "files" all of our day's information into our memory banks.

When I sleep well, I wake up and the world looks and feels fresh and inviting. I step out of bed with a spring in my step and can face anything the day will throw my way. But I also realize that there are times when I'm not going to get the sleep quota that I need, let alone want. What's essential then, is to try to get quality sleep for those precious hours; it may not be as much as I'd like, but it will still do the trick. So if I know I'm going to get short rations, I really "prep" for

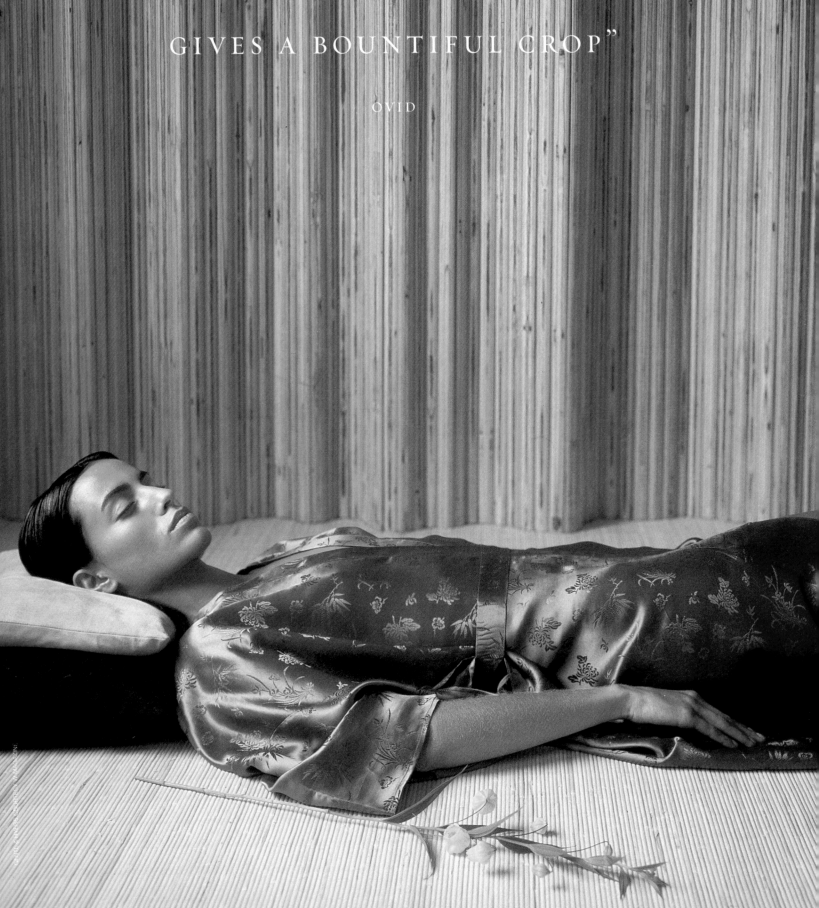

"TAKE A REST: A FIELD THAT HAS RESTED
GIVES A BOUNTIFUL CROP"

OVID

bed, to make it easier to drift off quickly and sleep deeply. It's not enough just to hit the pillow with my fingers crossed. Sometimes, as a treat, I'll book a massage late in the afternoon or early in the evening, especially if I've had a really tough day. I find that shiatsu massage, which focuses on releasing energy by applying pressure on strategic points throughout the body, is particularly good for shifting me right into a wonderful, healthy sleep mode.

Our bodies are ruled by biorhythm cycles that keep us alert or allow us to unwind. If I find that I'm getting sleepy, usually between 10 P.M. and 11 P.M., I try to catch that "sleep wave." If I fight it and stay up longer, I eventually start to panic: I've lost the wave and I know it's going to be much harder to get to sleep when I finally land in bed. Even if you haven't managed to get everything accomplished, I think it's better to leave it—and start afresh in the morning. The next morning you will feel renewed and ready to tackle the day.

MY GOLDEN RULES FOR GREAT SLEEP

DON'T EAT TOO LATE My absolute cut-off time for mealtime is 9 P.M., though 8 P.M. is preferable, and 7:30 is best of all. Better to go to bed hungry and eat a good breakfast than be kept awake by your body trying to process a late-night meal.

BECOME A FRESH AIR FIEND Stuffy rooms aren't conducive to great sleep because the oxygen level is lower. I keep the window wide open, even in winter, and snuggle under a warm comforter.

ENTER THE AROMA ZONE Lavender essential oil is a tried-and-tested sleep aid; I find a few drops on my pillow—or even a dab under my nose—fantastically soporific. Neroli, sandalwood, and geranium are effective on the pillow, too. (Neroli can be applied right on the skin, but the others are too potent for direct application.)

TUNE IN TO WHITE NOISE I keep a gizmo by my bed—the Heart and Sound Soother from The Sharper Image, see Resources—that offers a choice of background sounds that work to drown out other noises. I am sure I live on the noisiest street in Manhattan; there are garbage trucks, taxis, delivery trucks, and caterers' vans that seem to work 'round the clock. But my "white noise" machine helps block out the extraneous sound, soothing me with sounds of the ocean. I can visualize the waves rolling onto the beach, and I drift off. It's more soothing than counting sheep—sometimes I can't quite get them over the fence! If sound is still a problem, I use little wax earplugs (called "Quies"), which you can find in most pharmacies: small balls of wax you warm in your fingers, and place in your ears. They don't blot out every sound, but they do comfortably muffle enough so I feel as if I'm cocooned.

BATH-TO-BED ((See The Magic Bath, p.150) According to sleep experts, the warming effect of a bath on the brain improves deep, slow-wave sleep.

YOGA AND YAWN In the morning, I love my "Salutation to the Sun," a classic exercise that limbers you up and gets the energy flowing for the day. I do it quickly, because the speed gets my circulation going. But at night, I love what I call my "Salutation to the Moon"—the same exercise, but practiced much more slowly. It makes me feel calm and prepares me perfectly for bed.

SALUTATION TO THE MOON

1   Stand up tall with your feet together and arms at your side. Take a deep breath and as you exhale, bring your palms together in a "prayer" position.

2   Inhale. With your palms still together, gently stretch your arms up and back over your head. Allow your hips to push forward.

3   Exhale as you stretch your hands down toward your toes, with your palms toward the floor. Bending forward, place your hands next to your feet, palms on the floor. (You can bend your knees a bit if you need to.) Tuck your forehead in toward your knees.

4   Inhale and stretch your right leg straight back behind you as far as you can. Bend the right knee, lowering your hips close to the ground. Your hands should remain on either side of your feet as you stretch your head and look upward. Retain your breath.

5   Bring your left leg back to meet the right. Keep your arms straight and your body in a plank position on your toes, not dropping your hips or head. Hold for a few seconds as you stretch.

6   Exhale. Gently lower your knees to the floor, arms still extended in front of you. Shift your weight to your heels. Keeping as low to the ground as possible, slowly extend your body forward toward your hands.

7   Inhale as you slowly continue stretching by arching your back and looking up toward the ceiling. Your arms should be straight, close to your body, supporting your upper weight, and hips should be on the floor.

8   Exhale, tucking your toes under and raising your hips into an inverted V. Keep your hands flat and your elbows and knees straight.

9   Inhale. Bring your right foot forward and place it on the floor between the palms, dropping your left knee to the ground.

10   Exhale and bring your left foot forward and place it next to your right foot. Raise your hips and stretch them upward, keeping your hands on the floor (bend your knees slightly if you need to).

11   Inhale and slowly roll up, one vertebra at a time. Exhale and bring your hands together.

This is one round. Repeat, extending the opposite leg first.

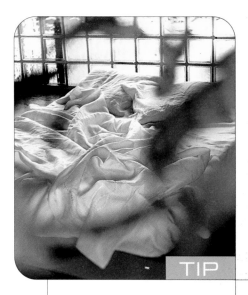

TIP

THE ART OF THE NAP

It's hard to find the time for a proper nap during the day, so I recommend the catnap: five minutes of "downtime" whenever and wherever you can. You can nap almost anywhere: in a doctor's waiting room, on the train, even a few minutes at your desk. Find a comfortable position, close your eyes, and take two or three deep breaths. It's a lot like a mini-meditation; you're not really asleep, just semiconscious. But all the same, it's extremely restorative; just shutting off the messages from your eyes is amazingly restful: our eyes focus and register, taking in so much information during the day that they deserve a break. And when your eyes are resting, your mind can, too.

BAN BAD NEWS FROM THE BEDROOM

"Sleep hygienists"—medical professionals who run clinics to help people conquer insomnia and sleep better—recommend you keep TV out of the bedroom. It's too addictive and with ninetysomething channels, you can't help worrying you're going to miss something. In particular, news and current affairs can be troublesome. They can make it harder to unwind and can actually disturb sleep patterns. According to experts, even reading the newspaper can have the same effect. Saving office work or bills for bed is a bad idea as well, because your mind will still be at work when your head is on the pillow.

Drink your milk. If I know sleep may be elusive, or if I'm not going to get my full quota, I turn to the old-fashioned savior—hot milk with honey. It always seems to work. I avoid caffeine after 4 p.m.-ish, because it keeps my mind buzzing long after my body's given up.

BECOME A MASKED WOMAN I can't live without my face-mask. It's so worn that I've actually asked my mother to copy it and make me a new one. Eye masks are fantastic for blocking out the light. The key is finding one that not only does the job, but is comfortable, too. Try before you buy; the elastic is often too tight (although you can snip it off and replace it with looser elastic).

I also love little eye pillows filled with sesame seeds. You can make your own, sewing together two rectangles of silk or cotton, about eight inches by four inches, and filling the pouch with sesame seeds. The weight of the seeds stops your eyelids from flickering, which is instantly restful. Another eye-calming trick is to rest the heels of your hands on your eyes for a few moments during the day, or place cold, wet cotton pads over the eyes during a catnap. Simply resting the eyes can make you feel like you've caught up on a valuable bit of sleep.

MAKE YOUR BED IRRESISTIBLE It's very important to me that my bed looks inviting, so when I walk through my room I can longingly think, "Boy, I can hardly wait to crawl inside." I have a comfy headboard to lean against and I love beautiful sheets because frankly, when you spend a third of your life in bed (as we do), great linen is a real investment. My favorite is Egyptian cotton. I am also a major pillow researcher: I've been to hotels and insisted, "You have to sell me this pillow"—and usually, they will. I have all sizes, from big French square pillows to little ones I can rest a book on. And I love those big, long, body-shaped pillows. If there's no live body next to you to cuddle, these pillows aren't a bad substitute!

LIQUID REFRESHMENT I hate waking up thirsty in the middle of the night, so I keep a pretty decanter of water and a glass by my bed. If you have to get up in the night for water, it interrupts the rhythm of your night.

DRESS FOR (SLEEP) SUCCESS I love to wear something beautiful to bed; if you'd do it for someone else, why not do it for yourself? Don't wait for someone to buy you fabulous nightwear—indulge yourself! I found some luscious, inexpensive silk satin pajamas in Bloomingdale's; they are cut like men's pajamas and are cool in summer, warm in winter. I have them in mint, white, and pink (and gave them to girlfriends for Christmas, too); I believe pale colors are more restful. (Although black negligees also have their place!)

LAUGHTER
IS THE BEST MEDICINE

The fastest way to take off ten years is to smile. Nothing communicates true beauty faster than laughter and smiling. When people ask me, "What are your top beauty tips?" I say, "Stand up straight and smile!" If you're considering a facelift, it's got to be worth trying these first!

When you laugh, you have a direct connection with the heart—yours and other people's. I learned the true power of a smile when, for five days, I had the job of hostessing and welcoming people from all over the world for an event. In the beginning it felt unnatural having a smile plastered on my face all the time. But when I saw the relief people felt upon being welcomed with a big warm smile, I too was won over. Arriving from Israel, Japan, Australia, and all over the world, the guests came through the door of the huge hotel feeling disorientated after their long trip. A smile connected us, and they gravitated toward me. It warmed my heart as I saw them light up, and the energy we felt was tangible. That's what a smile can do.

In New York City, in particular, people smile far too rarely. After my experience hostessing, I started noticing as I walked along Fifth Avenue that so many really attractive women in their forties, fifties, and over were carrying the weight of the world on their faces, causing frown lines between the eyes, wrinkles on the forehead, and downturned lips. After a certain age, you have the face you have earned; how you feel about your life is written there for all to see. But whenever you smile, it defies gravity; everything goes upward in a flash. I have friends who obsess about the imperfection of certain body parts—eyes, noses, whatever—but all of that blends together when you smile. Suddenly, in a smile, you see the essence of a person—and the realization of their potential beauty.

I constantly try to remind myself of something I once read: that the more serious you are, the further you are away from your true self. That has always struck a chord with me. We cannot control everything that goes on in our lives, but laughter is connected with flexibility, with an ability to roll with the changes.

We have to plug into this universal humor when life is out of control. Recently, my daughter said something to me that made me burst out laughing. I had been complaining to her about leaving the soap "glued" to an impossibly difficult place to retrieve. She lifted one eyebrow and ironically replied, "Mom, pick your battles." You can't win everything, and that's where the laughter comes in. Sometimes, we have to remind ourselves of the joys in life. It can be as simple as enhancing our desk with a photograph of a child or our parents smiling back at us. Just one look at that photo, in the middle of some heavy-duty stress, can be all it takes to remember the joy.

As children, laughter was never far away. That's why it's so important to stay in touch with the child within each of us. We still are that child—a sweet and tender person—and it is she who gives us our sense of fun. And what is the point of life without fun?

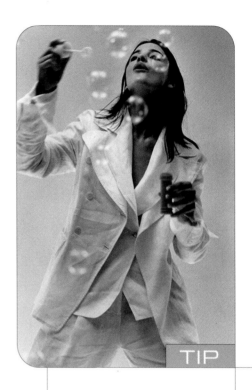

TIP

SILLY STUFF
For instant fun and laughter, try:
charades
Pictionary
Twister (the older you are, the funnier this gets—believe me)
kite-flying
old scrapbooks
outdoor games and sports
karaoke
children
bubbles
stuffed toys
funny movies
pets

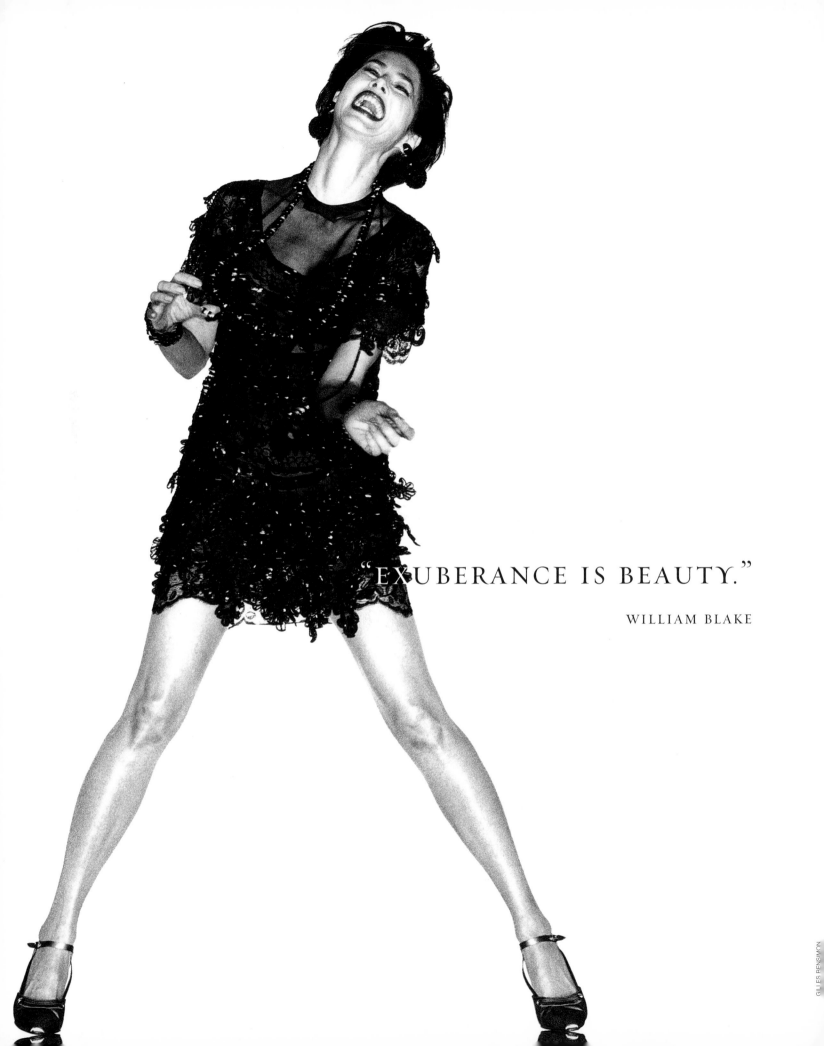

"EXUBERANCE IS BEAUTY."

WILLIAM BLAKE

YOU'VE GOT TO LAUGH: THE FACTS Scientists are now confirming: laughter really is the best medicine. According to Dr. William F. Fry of Stanford University Medical School, laughter triggers the release of the antibody immunoglobulin A, which boosts the immune system. Medical and psychological research papers have shown that fun keeps you fit: A good laugh acts like a sort of internal aerobics, working the muscles of the heart and upper body, stimulating the nerves, and improving the way the body uses oxygen. There is now even such a thing as "mirth medicine," pioneered by a man named Norman Cousins. He was suffering from a crippling disease from which he had a 1-in-500 chance of recovery. To brighten his day, he started watching Marx Brothers films and discovered that the pleasure of a single film gave him at least two hours of pain-free sleep. Inspired, he checked out of the hospital and into a hotel room—where he laughed himself back to health. Today, Dr. Patch Adams, a "doctor clown," plans to open a "silly hospital" in Virginia, helping to make patients better by prescribing laughter: funny films, games, and toys. And in the United Kingdom, in 1991, a Laughter Clinic was established in the Birmingham public hospital.

SHEER INDULGENCES

Sheer indulgences may seem like luxuries but they can also be real lifesavers. I believe that taking the time to do something rejuvenating is a life-extender. Indulgence is as much about taking time as spending money. Time for yourself extends the quality, and potentially the length, of your life.

So seize the day, the hour, the moment. We spend our lives planning for tomorrow, often postponing pleasure, perhaps out of some misplaced guilt or a sense that somehow we don't deserve a treat. But if we don't take care of ourselves now, tomorrow may never come. If you're a businessperson or are taking care of a family, you're usually at the bottom of the priority list. Sheer indulgence is about putting yourself first. What you'll discover when you dip into these indulgences is that they can bring back the joy in your life. Suddenly, after taking a moment for yourself, work doesn't seem so difficult. Problems may not disappear, but their importance fades. It's all about rebalancing.

GET A MASSAGE This tops my list, but it's not for everyone; for my mother, massage is undesirable because she's from a generation that is not as at ease with someone touching her. Indulgence for her is about a new bottle of perfume or a silk scarf or taking the time to window shop.

TAKE A COOKING CLASS to master your favorite cuisine. Then invite a friend over to show off your new skills!

INVEST IN BEAUTIFUL STATIONERY and a special writing pen to create your own personalized notes.

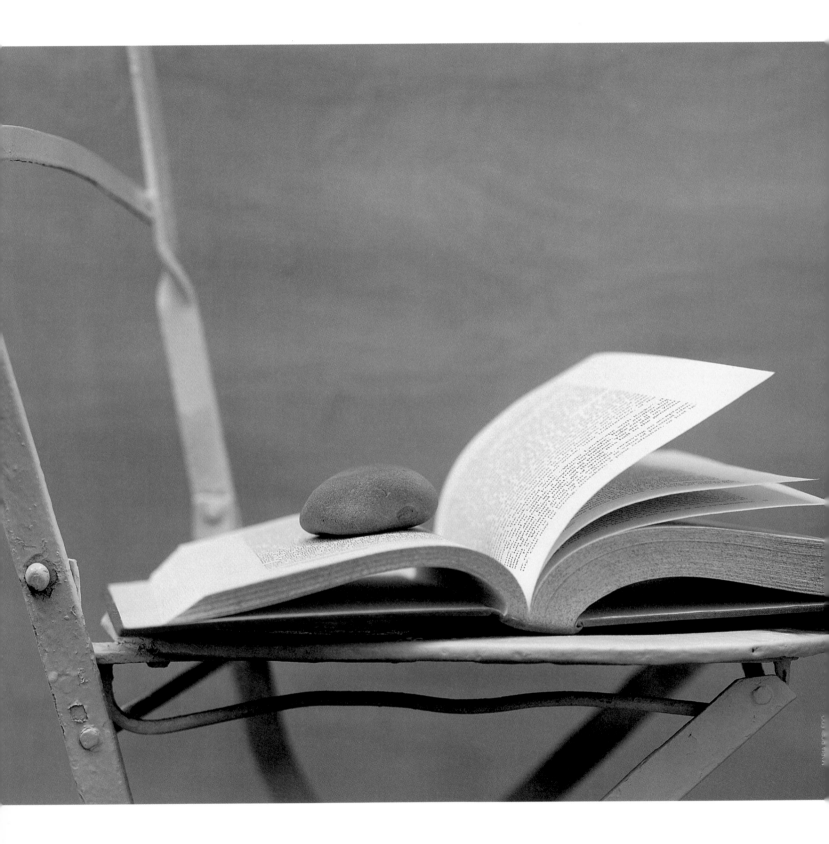

DIVE INTO A BOOK that you've always wanted to read instead of a pile of papers. Treat yourself to a hardcover!

LEARN A LANGUAGE or brush up on one you took in school. Perhaps this will fuel your fantasy of traveling abroad.

INDULGE IN A TRULY LUXURIOUS BATH (See p. 150 for my Magic Bath). This is one of my favorites!

BUY YOURSELF FLOWERS (If we wait for a man to buy us flowers, we may have to wait a very long time!) An orchid, especially, is a beautiful indulgence—and because it lasts an amazingly long time, it can work out to be less expensive than cut flowers in the long run.

TRY A WONDERFUL NEW PERFUME There is something luxurious about experimenting with a new scent and deciding if it enhances the new you.

TREAT YOURSELF TO DELICIOUS NEW PILLOWCASES AND SHEETS How wonderful is it to tuck yourself into bed after a long day, warmly wrapped in crisp, new sheets? Total luxury.

DIG IN YOUR GARDEN Smell and feel the rich earth and watch your efforts change and grow each day. I became so passionate with my garden in L.A. that I actually found myself digging by flashlight one evening!

TAKE A MUSIC APPRECIATION COURSE or learn calligraphy, pottery, or oil painting. A friend of mine goes to opera classes where she learns about the great composers. I took singing classes for a while, not because I wanted to become the next Beverly Sills but because it was such fun to be able to sing the songs I love.

HAVE A PEDICURE even if nobody else is going to see your feet. I gave my sister Darilyn a "beauty weekend" in New York. She is not into the "beauty thing" at all. But she had such an unexpected pleasure from looking down at her toes all painted red, wiggling and admiring them in her hiking sandals, that we're going to do it again!

VISIT A SPA FOR THE DAY Many towns now have a day spa. Book yourself in for a half-day and discover seaweed wraps, salt scrubs, aromatherapy, reflexology. Give yourself a treat—maybe a few times a year. Ask for a visit for your birthday or for Mother's Day, instead of requesting another ornament that needs dusting.

All of this is about opening more windows to happiness.

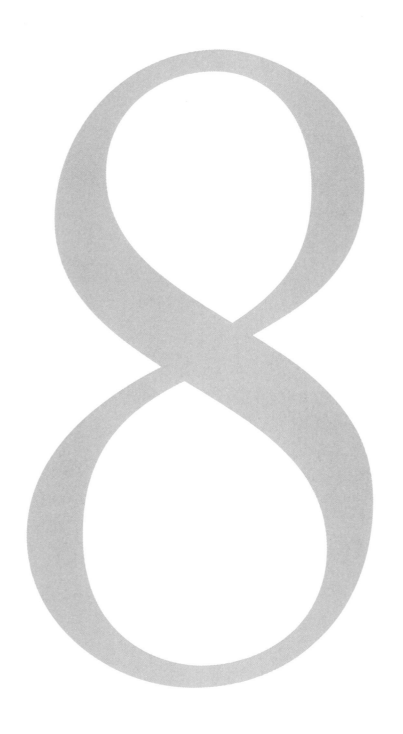

HEALTHY MIND, HEALTHY YOU

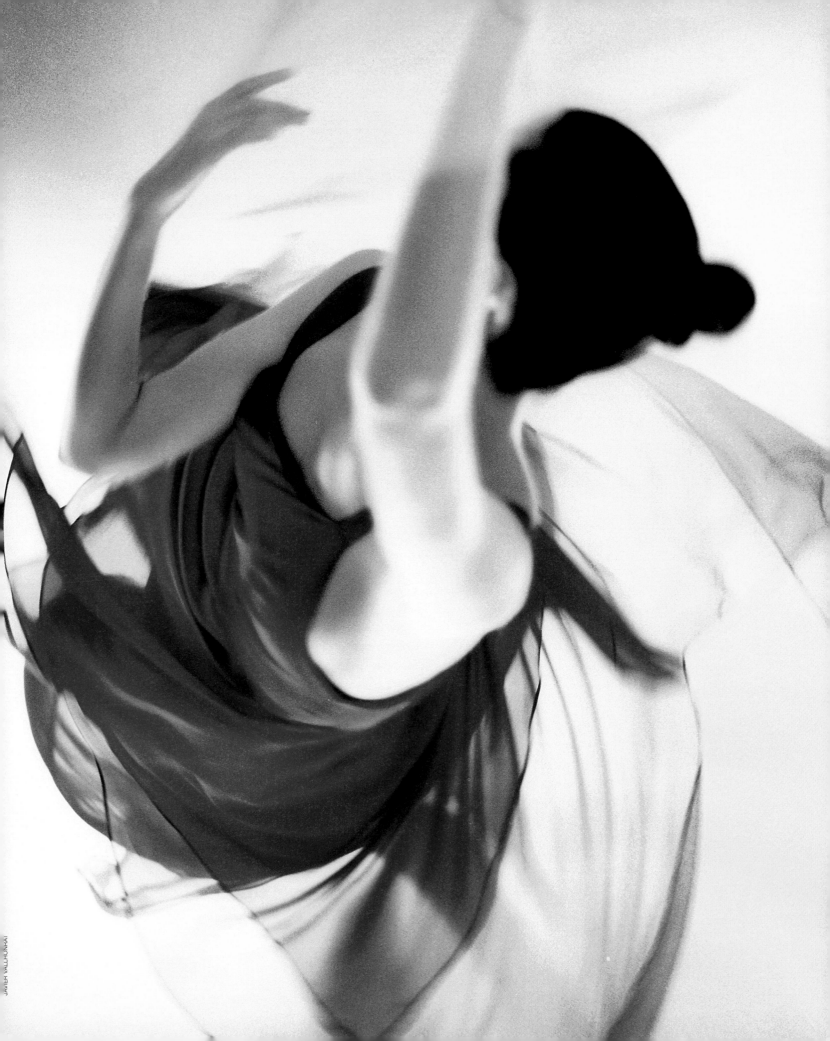

FIND YOUR PASSION

We work, work, work, work, work. We know what our duties are. Now it is time to find what our passions are. Our passions nurture us. Our passions light the fire within. Spending half an hour a day or an hour or two each week fulfilling our passions enables us to get through the things we *have* to do. Our duties may drain us, but our passions give us the opportunity to renew ourselves. Because when we create a passion in our life, we are refueled; re-energized to tackle the work, the people, and the challenges of life.

You know all those excuses we have about not having enough time? If you spend time on what you are passionate about, it will save you time in the long run—and give you the energy and inspiration to get the most out of life. If you have a passion, it can really help you through the tough times—times of loss, fear, stress, can't pay the bills, or are facing a major life challenge. If you have developed a passion, you have a place inside yourself where you can retreat, cuddle up, and be healed.

Ask yourself: What excites me? Be logical. Be crazy. Think about what makes sense and nonsense to you. My mother, in her sixties, developed a passion for doll making. She still works full-time running doctors' offices, but when she comes home she rejuvenates her spirit by creating beautiful dolls from scratch: bodies, heads, clothes. The best part for her is giving them away. She is fueled by the magical expression on the faces of the children as they hold their treasured handmade doll for the first time.

Many women have what I call a "too-good-to-forget box"—a place to tuck away newspaper clippings, magazines articles, great ideas. If you're looking for inspiration to kick start a passion, start there.

A simple interest can eventually become a passion—so if there's nothing you feel passionate about, at least start with a healthy interest. Friends have said to me, "I'm good at many things but not great at anything." We're talking fun, not function here; soul, not necessarily skill. And, who knows . . . you may find you're not half bad!

Following your passion is *exciting*. I had no idea, for instance, that I would ever write a book. Yet, here I am, passionate about sharing my ideas and being able to talk with women through these pages. I wanted to share what I've learned and what I believe with other women. Out of this desire grew a business. The passion I feel for what I am doing gives me incredible energy: I can work fourteen, sixteen, eighteen hours a day or get straight off a plane and hit the ground running simply because I love what I'm doing so much. I think this kind of passion is infectious.

In India, there is a wonderful word—*rasa*—the inner appetite for life, the "juice." If you use the *rasa* up without replenishing it, you become "dry"; you do things without animation and there is no inner joy. That is the beginning of the end, the downward spiral, and it should ring alarm bells. At various points in my

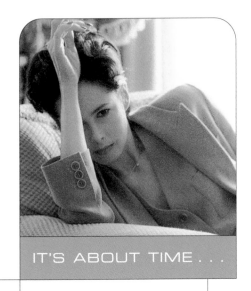

IT'S ABOUT TIME . . .

. . . to accept that a healthy mind means a healthy you. At midlife, we experience infinite freedom. Liberated from the hang-ups of youth and the day-to-day responsibility of caring for children or climbing the career ladder, it's time to find our passion. Follow the joy. Enrich our very souls. Discover the things that give meaning to life and answer some of its biggest questions. Helping to keep us balanced and grounded in a hectic, crazy world.

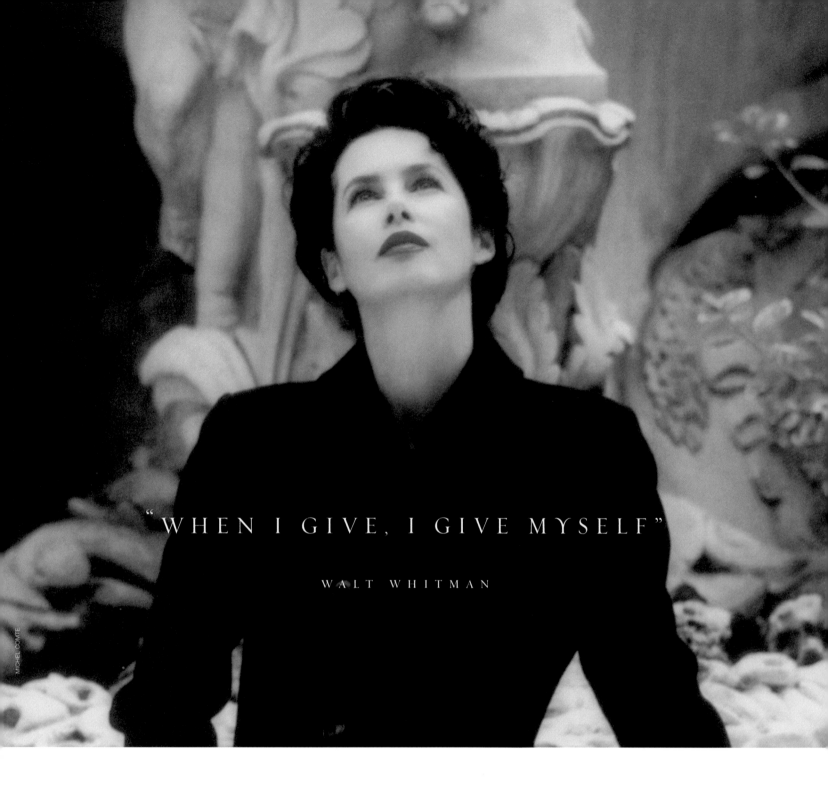

"WHEN I GIVE, I GIVE MYSELF"

WALT WHITMAN

life, I have met women who are near the bottom of that spiral; they are scared, realizing they've used everything up and are hurtling toward disaster, heading for a breakdown. They are searching for something to be passionate about, to relight the fire, but they have nothing left. It's like trying to start a fire by rubbing two sticks together, but in slow motion and without conviction. It just doesn't work. So find your passion now, incorporate it into your life, and make some time to celebrate and nurture it. The joy of building your passion will fuel the fire of life and keep it blazing.

BELONGING

Looking beautiful on the outside is worth nothing if we feel an emptiness in our souls. Unfortunately, in this fast-paced, helter-skelter world, it is easy to lose our sense of belonging. That loss of connection has an impact on our health, on our well-being and on how we look. It can make us feel old before our time.

The answer is to reconnect. As soon as you are part of something bigger, you no longer feel alone. And this, quite simply, is a firm foundation for happiness and good health. Studies are now revealing that the more friends and connections you have, the greater the variety of your social contact, and the better your health.

I was fascinated to find out about a study at Carnegie Mellon University in Pittsburgh; they exposed 276 people to cold viruses and found that those with fewer links to family, friends, and community were more likely to become ill. Other studies at Cornell University have shown that people who volunteer suffer fewer illnesses and live longer than those who don't.

So linking with any community or any group—from a charity organization to a baking club, from a sewing bee to a reading group—is life-giving. It gives you a feeling of value and belonging, enhancing your sense of well-being and even your general health.

I know the importance of belonging from my own life. After the loss of my husband, home, security, and peace of mind, I tried to work through the pain and get back on my feet. I volunteered at Cedars-Sinai Hospital to spend time in what was called "play therapy" with children undergoing cancer treatment. The children ranged in age from two to twelve and I took care of them while they waited to have their chemotherapy. Trying to comfort and entertain children suffering through such an obviously painful and traumatic time was a challenge. Sometimes, members of their families were also struggling with conflicting emotions about all the focus being on the sick child; they too needed attention. So it was important for me to be involved with the entire family. Over time, I found that as I helped others, I really helped myself. I was so focused on healing, giving, loving, and sharing around me, I forgot about my own difficulties. I realized that my problems were not the only ones, not the biggest or the most devastating problems in the world and that my pain, though personal and crushing, was a universal emotion, part of the fabric of life. Such revelations gave me perspective and strength and helped me survive *my* difficult time.

There are, of course, countless ways to volunteer. Mentoring is another way to give back to the community by helping young people realize their potential (see Resources). One of the things that sometimes discourages us, however, is worrying that we don't have enough talent or time to contribute anything significant. First of all, we all have talent. We each have our experiences, goodness, and willingness to give. This is the gift of ourselves and as for time, most charities and community groups are happy to have any help, for however short a time—even just once a month or on a project-by-project basis.

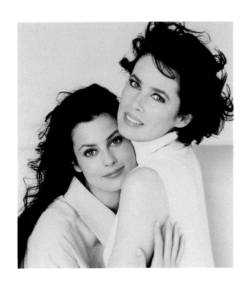

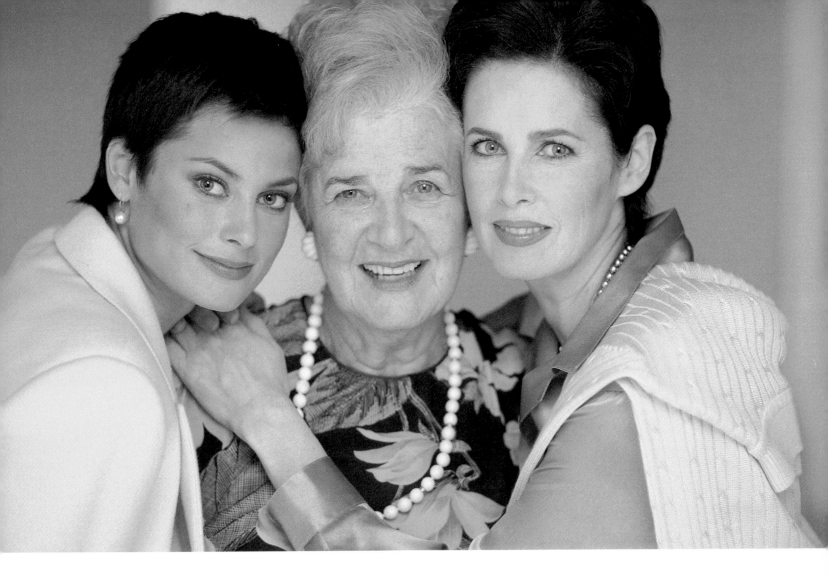

Three generations: Ryan, Terry, and Dayle

What is also crucial, I believe, is to strengthen relationships between the generations. In midlife, we're perfectly poised to bridge the generational gap. At forty, we are "elders" and yet still "youngsters"—with value. There is a great deal we can teach younger generations and a great deal we can do to help older people.

We still have plenty to learn from our elders. Don't forget about the old people in your own family or take them for granted. Sit down with a parent, a grandmother, or an aunt and share family stories and legends; ask about their experiences and memories. Don't let your rich history disappear when they do. My sister and I love to listen to our father's stories. He has so many riveting tales about the tank he commandeered as a nineteen year old in Holland during the Second World War. My sister Darilyn wrote down all his reminiscences, making a little book of his memories, which she presented to him. He was thrilled. Older people, like all of us, love having someone who will listen to them. It lets them hold onto and share life's most special moments and keeps them feeling young, as well. And, lucky for us, it gives insights into who we are, where we came from, and where we might be heading.

Whatever you give, you get back many-fold; giving is the ultimate investment in others and yourself.

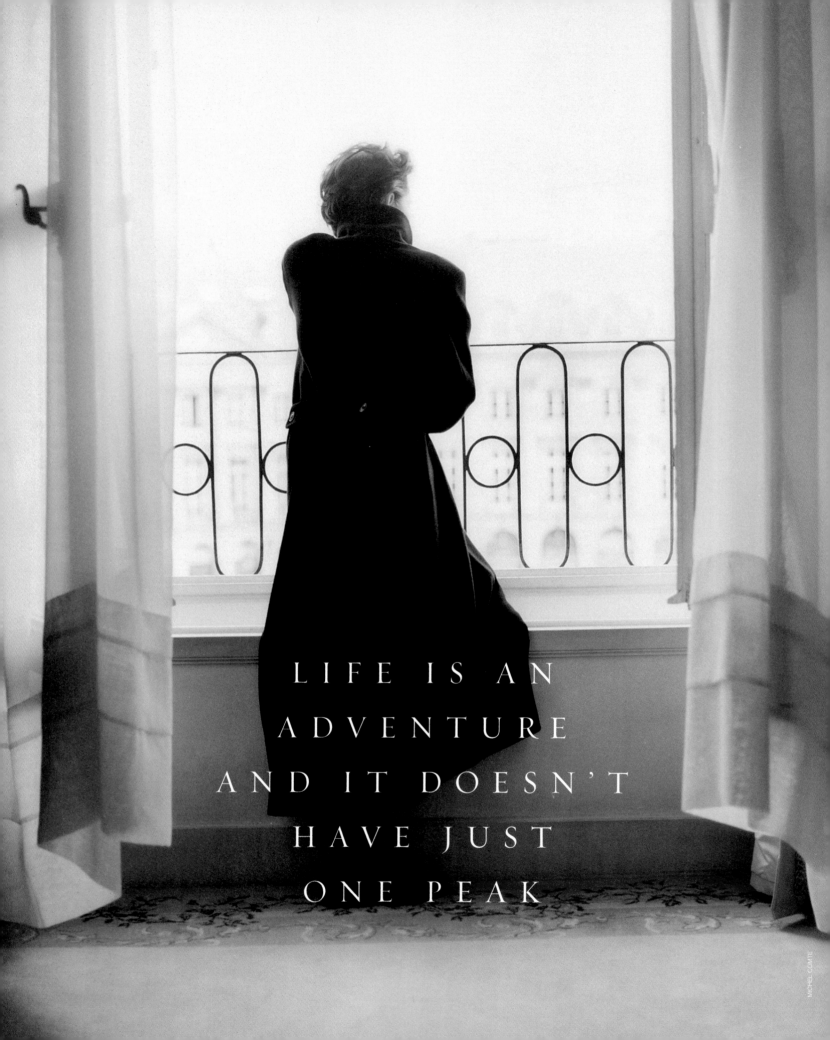

LIFE IS AN
ADVENTURE
AND IT DOESN'T
HAVE JUST
ONE PEAK

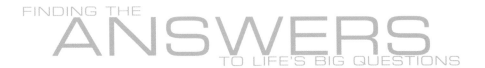
I cannot imagine life without a sense of spirituality. I don't mean religion; I mean a sense of something greater than my own smaller wants and needs, a feeling of connection with those around me, and a belief that everything and everyone has a purpose—that there is a divine plan. It is really important for me to have a sense of this as I move through life, because it places all of my joys, my difficulties, my heartaches, and my dreams into proportion; I can allow the magic to enter my life. This "magic" opens up possibilities to manage the things that are beyond my control and brings a sense of joy to all I do and see.

Being spiritual doesn't necessarily mean going to this church or that temple. It can be those things, but it doesn't have to be. Religion is more about the way you organize and prefer to express your spirituality, but the practice of spirituality is as varied as we are individuals. Everyone's religious beliefs should be respected; this is how people decide to access the spiritual side of their life—which is an intensely personal decision. It is knowing when to surrender and accept and when to use self-effort to change what needs to be changed.

My feeling of spirituality involves a sense of communion with all things: nature, mankind, the universe. Through this sense of spirituality, I believe I can begin to answer some of life's big questions. My advice: Follow the joy. I can't say it often enough: Joy will steer you toward what is right for you. What are the things that make you feel uplifted? What makes your heart sing? What gives you strength and comfort?

At midlife, we are better prepared to look for answers to life's big questions. By the time we reach our forties, we have lived long enough to have wisdom to draw from, and yet we still have so much ahead of us. We want (and demand) a quality of life we may not have been ready to experience or appreciate at a younger age. Meditation, prayer, and contemplation are tools we can use to access those answers. Meditation in itself is quite magical. As passive as it may appear, meditation can involve moments of great activity; tremendous insights can come to you while meditating. If I have a problem with somebody or an argument that isn't resolved, I will often take that problem into a meditation, sit with it, and wait and see what comes up. I may not find the answer right away, but often it will come to me later in the day (for more on meditation, see p. 172). Prayer is also a powerful tool to gather strength, express gratitude, or simply to give thanks. Whether you're meditating, praying, or contemplating, simply accessing your spiritual side is easier, away from the frenzy of day-to-day life.

It is this day-to-day work on ourselves that takes us to the place where we can see and hear more clearly. The answers to life's big questions may not reveal themselves instantly, in a blinding flash. Instead, working on the self can be a little like peeling an onion. It's often a subtle step-by-step process; you peel away one layer, then the next, slowly seeing and hearing more clearly. Then there's a revelation; suddenly the way you perceive your life is quite different as you discover new insights and inspirations.

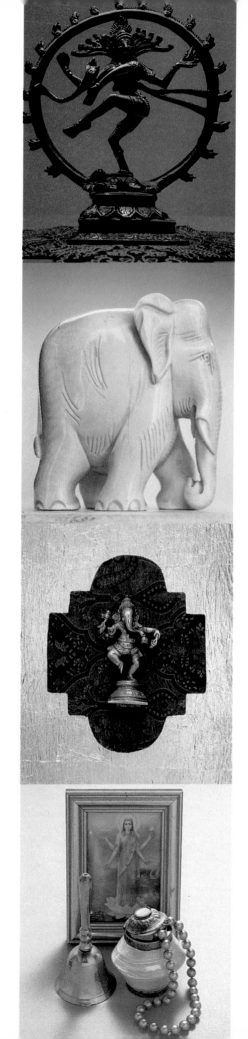

ZEN
AND THE ART OF DISHWASHING

Meditation, from the Greek word "to be mindful," can seem too mysterious and esoteric; in other words, too wacky to be part of day-to-day life. Even when women are curious about meditation, it often feels too foreign for them to know how or where to start. When we have so little time, why do we need yet another activity that's going to eat into our schedule? When we have responsibilities, we do not want to give up our time unless there is going to be a valuable payback.

Well, that's exactly what meditation delivers. You need less sleep, which is just as well, because you may need to get up a little earlier to do it! You have more patience for the ups and downs of the day's roller-coaster. You respond to things less emotionally. Do it regularly and your concentration and focus will become better and you will achieve balance in your life. That's a *promise*. Meditation also delivers the insights you need for problem solving. And there's yet another great reason to meditate: Researchers at the University of Massachusetts Medical Center have discovered that daily meditation boosts the level of melatonin, a hormone that fights free radical damage and minimizes the effects of aging.

Meditation is simple, natural, and easy. It doesn't require any equipment, tons of time, or special clothing. You don't have to embrace some new religion or run off to a Tibetan monastery. Although you may not realize it, you meditate already: When you concentrate so fully that you lose yourself in what you are doing, you are basically meditating. Meditation is a form of concentration.

Our lives are spent focused on what's going on outside of ourselves: dealing with the car that won't start, lost keys, the FedEx that never arrives, getting a bill we weren't expecting, and that broken toilet. With all that stuff going on, life becomes more about the world and less about you. That's why it's so important to make that 180-degree turn inwards, to restore balance. "Rebalancing" on a regular basis makes the inner you bigger and puts the outer world back into proportion, so you can better deal with the weeds, daily dishes, IRS, and that annoying neighbor. It is your time to get in touch with yourself. Your time for you.

Not only will meditation vastly improve the quality of your day-to-day life, it could extend it, too. Research now shows that this tension-banishing technique, practiced regularly, can help control a wide range of complaints, from headaches to asthma, eczema to PMS, hypertension, and even heart attacks. (One U.K. study of meditation and relaxation training for men and women at risk of coronary disease found that after four years, not only did the meditating group reduce their blood pressure readings, but also experienced fewer symptoms of heart disease, and a lower number of deaths from heart attacks.)

How often have I heard the excuse, "I don't have time to meditate"? But everyone can make the time. If you have a family, a busy house to deal with, or a long commute in the morning, you might want to set your alarm just ten minutes earlier so that you can have that quiet time for yourself to meditate before your day begins. You can also meditate in bite-sized chunks: when you're walking, or at your desk, or even while washing the dishes.

USING SOUND, SCENT, AND SPACE TO HELP YOU FOCUS

My friend Jo, who lives in London, has a beautiful, small brass bell that she rings when she starts and finishes a project. She searched for a long time for her bell, in thrift markets and antique shops and took great joy in finding one with exactly the right sweet sound. You can use a bell—or chimes (like my friend Michele)—to start and finish a meditation; these are tools that help you go within. It also brings a sense of ceremony to what you are about to do.

Where I was staying in India, there was a Chinese gong that was struck each morning and at the end of each day. It had an exquisite, calming resonance that lingered in the courtyard, tingling deep inside the body. Certain chimes, bells, and some musical instruments resonate, and by following the resonation, it can lead you deeper within. (It's fun to find your own.) I play a tape of sitar music when I meditate. The sitar has a very relaxing, repetitive sound that also draws you inward when you follow it, making meditating that much easier.

I also have a special incense that I burn when I meditate, called Blue Pearl. Some of the Indian incenses are too sweet and soapy for me, but this one has a beautiful scent and reminds me so much of India. When my friends visit they often comment how much they love the way my house smells. You might want to find a special incense that you burn only when you're meditating. Over time, the smell of the incense or the sound of your bell/gong/tape can help you take a shortcut, to speed you on your "inner journey" and quickly turn you inward again so that you become more relaxed and focused. It becomes your own ritual.

It helps to meditate in the same place every time. Eventually, you build up a certain energy in that spot so that you can simply glide right into meditation by being there. Try to pick a space in your home where there isn't too much traffic and use that as your meditation area. I have a little shelf with special objects that help with my meditation and make it easier for me to turn inward: a quartz crystal, an amethyst, some beachcombed stones that I think are special, a bell, a fresh flower, a delicious-smelling little sandalwood carving of the Indian elephant deity Ganesh, "the remover of all obstacles." (We all need those in our lives!) Once you've found your corner, place a few objects there that help you connect with your heart —perhaps a picture of a child you love, or a souvenir of a magical trip.

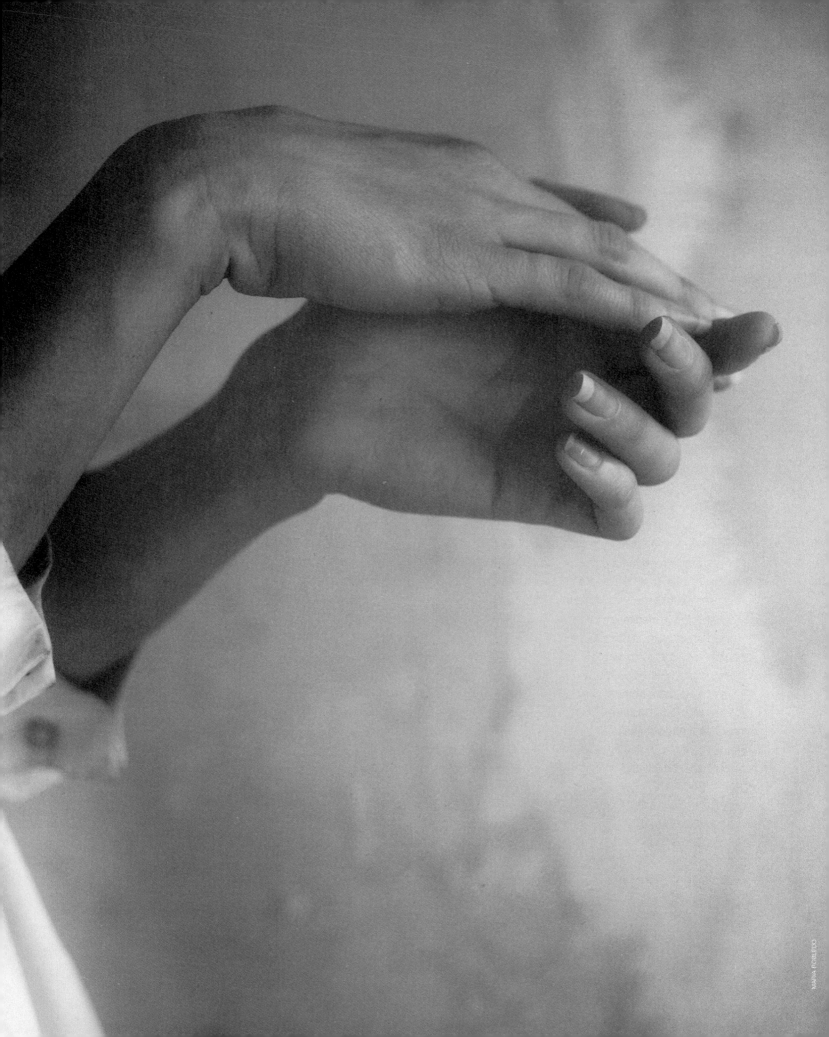

DAILY MEDITATION   For me, the hours before 7 A.M. and after 6 P.M. are the best to meditate. I feel I have stolen this time from my day. I live on a very noisy midtown street in Manhattan, so the morning is a quieter time, before the hum of the city begins. Being up earlier than most people in the city makes me feel that whatever I am doing at this time is special.

Here is how I meditate. These are not hard-and-fast rules: Do what works for you, at the time that's best for you.

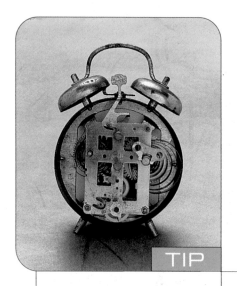

TIP

- Wear loose, light clothing. Try to wear the same clothes each time, saving them only for your meditations.
- Meditate in the same place each day.
- Remove your shoes and sit cross-legged, preferably on a piece of wool fabric or blanket (this helps hold the energy), placed on a comfortable cushion.
- Put your thumbs and forefingers together and gently place them on your knees or in your lap.
- Close your eyes. Sit with your spine as straight as you can (imagine a line going from the base of your spine to the top of your head).
- Take a deep breath. Go ahead, take another.
- Gently follow the breath. Follow it in and then slowly out. Focus on the space between the in breath and the out breath.
- Keep focusing on the breath, and continue for ten to fifteen minutes or until you feel ready.

NOTE: If you find yourself thinking about your laundry or bills you have to pay, don't panic. Just acknowledge your thoughts and gently return your focus to the in breath and the out breath.

REMINDER: Go slow. Be gentle with yourself. Don't get discouraged; like anything new, meditation takes a bit of practice. But the rewards, over time, are extraordinary. At the beginning, set aside just ten to fifteen minutes. You can increase the time as you go along. Each time you meditate it may be different; sometimes you feel as if you've emerged from a deep sleep, other times it feels like nothing at all has happened. I had amazing results the first time I meditated and felt a perceptible change in the balance of my life within a week. At other times, it seemed as if nothing happened, but I kept at it.

Today, meditation gives me a new perspective on my day right away.

Take note of how different your day is when you meditate from days when you don't.

When a friend recently asked what meditation does for me, I explained that it puts a little distance between me and the world—that little bit of extra perspective allowing me to see life more clearly. When we're in the middle of dressing a wriggling kid or trying to pull off a high-pressure business deal, we usually don't have any space to step back. But every time we do step back to view the bigger picture, it gives us more room to negotiate. Meditation gives us that little bit of extra space. It cushions the stress of our lives, so that we have the room to really observe what is going on. Meditation also helps you to be aware of the present moment, instead of being stuck in the past or anxious for the future. It slows life down. You've given yourself the gift of more time.

HEAVEN
SCENT

Scent is one of the most immediate ways I know to lift my mood. If I'm feeling tired, a spritz of eucalyptus or peppermint into the air picks me right up. A fragrant bouquet of Casablanca lilies on my living room table welcomes me home as I walk through the door. (Lilies are fantastically long-lasting, continuing to give off their delicious scent right up to the time you have to toss them out.) When I lived in L.A., I grew wild lavender and geraniums in my garden. Just stepping outside and taking in their fragrance was enough for me to start to unwind.

Once upon a time, of course, our noses were incredibly important; they warned of approaching sabre-toothed tigers, helped locate ripe berries, even signaled the perfect mate. When we are asleep, our sense of smell is the only sense that stays wide awake. Without it, our sense of taste all but disappears. But most of us neglect our sense of smell. Helen Keller, whose own nose was so acute that she could sense impending rain, described smell as the "fallen angel" of our senses. Today, we're assaulted by odors of pollution, garbage, stale air, and smoke, so it's no wonder we spend much of our time trying to cut ourselves off from the world of smells. I believe our sense of smell is like a muscle; just by using it, you'll train yourself to enhance the joy you get out of life.

Smells are processed in the forebrain, the part that deals with instincts and urges. Long-term memory is stored in the forebrain, too. Smell and memory overlap, therefore, and are later retrieved as a single experience. Recapturing the scent of a loved one can flood you with memories you may have forgotten; through the sense of smell, you can recapture the essence of a person—a powerful experience. Smells can transport you instantly through space and time. If I smell Guerlain's Vetiver, for instance, it can literally make me weak in the knees. At home, I burn an incense from Ganeshpuri, an ancient sacred valley in India that I visited—and I'm right back there, in a second. If I catch a whiff of a scent I've loved at certain times in my life —like Joy or L'Air du Temps—it's as if I have traveled back in time in a flash, to a vacation I had or a city I visited at another time in my life.

You can also use fragrance to change the atmosphere in a room. If there's been an argument or if you move into a home or an office where the atmosphere simply feels wrong, you can purify the air with incense—or, as the Native Americans do, by lighting a sage "smudge stick." It cleanses the air and shifts the energy. (I moved into an office recently that nobody had wanted to use. Burning some incense seemed to change the atmosphere, clearing it out. Now people don't want to leave!)

Today, scientists are finally waking up to the power of smell. In one study at New York's Sloan Kettering Memorial Hospital, anxiety levels were measured in patients undergoing MRI (Magnetic Resonance Imaging) scans, used to diagnose life-threatening illnesses. MRIs require perfect stillness in a confined

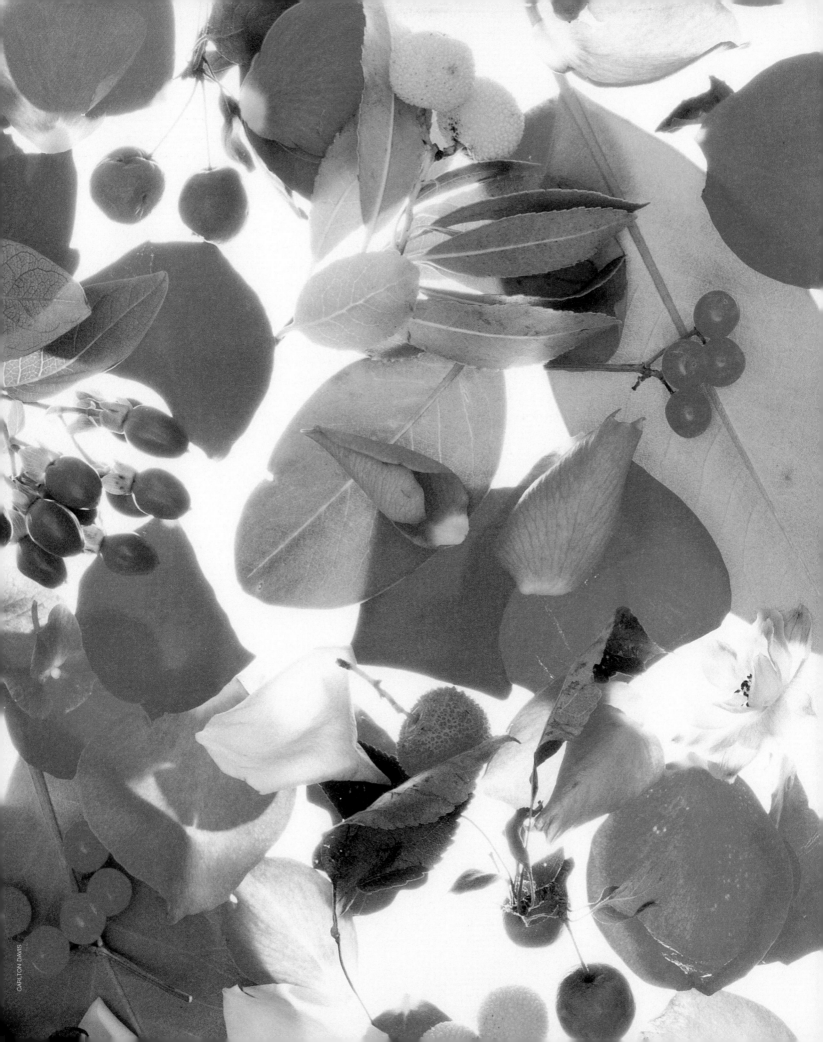

TIP

FROM STRENGTH
TO STRENGTH

Different strengths of fragrance last for varying lengths of time.

• Parfum/perfume: the richest, most intense of all, contains 20 percent fragrance and endures on the skin for four to six hours. (Remember: just a little goes a long way.)

• Eau de Parfum: 10 to 15 percent fragrance elements; lasts four to five hours.

• Eau de Toilette: 5 to 12 percent fragrance, lasts two to four hours.

• Eau Fraîche: around 3 percent perfume, lasts for around two hours.

• Eau de Cologne: 2 to 3 percent perfume, lingers on the skin for approximately two hours.

• Body lotion: lasts from three to eight hours. If you literally "layer" fragrance—using a scented bath product, then a body lotion or powder, with a spritz of fragrance as a finale—the result, surprisingly, isn't overpowering; instead, as the body heats and cools during the day, the various fragrance layers "come alive," allowing your fragrance to last and last.

space for up to an hour at a time. Often the strain is too much, so the expensive scan must be redone or cut short before results are achieved. But when patients sniffed vanilla—that warm, nurturing, Mom's-apron smell—they experienced 63 percent less panic than usual. Another scientific test (carried out by psychologist William December of the University of Cincinnati and Raj Parasuraman of Catholic University in Washington, D.C.) conclusively revealed that a whiff of peppermint or lily of the valley was highly effective at relieving the tedium of a dull job. In Japan, such research is being put into action: Peppermint or lemon fragrances are wafted through airshafts into some offices, to keep the workforce alert and efficient.

One thing is certain: Although in theory we can discern over 1,000 different smells, most of us have lazy noses. It might not seem important to rediscover the joy of smell, but all these little life-enhancers add up, like stringing pearls one by one to make a necklace. So take time to smell the roses—and fresh-baked cakes, newly laundered sheets, and thawing earth.

GREAT WAYS TO FRAGRANCE YOUR LIFE

CANDLES Some of my favorite scents are from Banana Republic (their Casablanca Lily is as close to the real thing as you can get), Aveda, Rigaud (from France), and Diptyque (their cinnamon candle is wonderful at Christmas). I also like to simmer a pan of water with a few cinnamon sticks and some cloves in it, for an instant Yuletide atmosphere. Light bulb oil rings, which let the fragrance seep out until it's filled the entire house, are great; my favorite fragrance for this is tuberose, which reminds me of the many flowers and garlands that abound in India.

POTPOURRI I'm not a big a fan of potpourri in general; so much of it looks like colored wood shavings, with a synthetic scent. Two exceptions are Agraria's Bitter Orange potpourri and Santa Maria Novella's potpourri (see Resources). The latter is made by monks in Florence from an ancient recipe and smells deliciously of cloves and spices. It's a very cleansing, almost medicinal scent, although it took me a bit of time to appreciate it fully.

ROOM SPRAYS I don't love commercial air fresheners—which are very synthetic-smelling. Instead I find mine at natural food stores. They are simply water sprays with essential oils; you can create your own, with a plant mister and some aromatherapy oils, and spritz into the air whenever it (or you) needs refreshing.

FRAGRANCE Fragrance is a wonderful way to get in touch with your feminine side. I first noticed the power of fragrance when I was five years old, observing my mother dabbing it behind her ears and wrists. I still love to see the thrill she gets receiving a new perfume. The fastest way for my mother to feel totally luxurious is to splash on her new gift.

I wear Fracas, fresh and floral for day, and Shalimar, sexy and exotic for nighttime. I've been a Fracas fan for so long now that occasionally I will stop

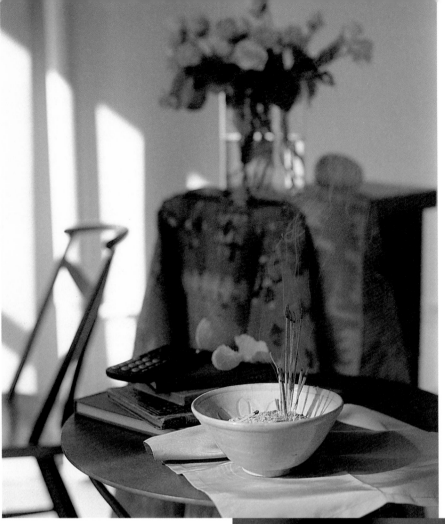

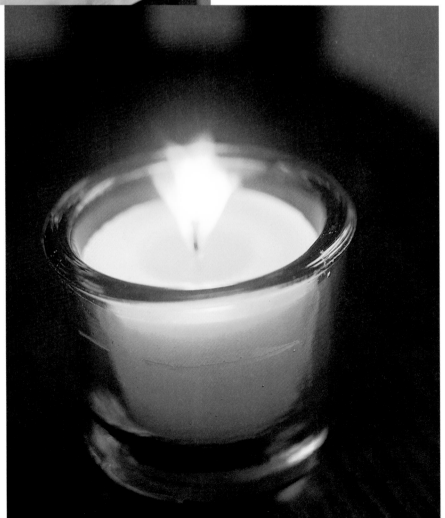

wearing it for a few days, so that I can have the pleasure of experiencing it again; sometimes, you just have to give your nose a rest! Another favorite fragrance is Penhaligon's Lily of the Valley (my birth flower). I prefer fragrances that are very individual. People will often ask me, "What are you wearing?" rather than just, "Oh, you're wearing X." It adds a little mystery. Another one of my great pleasures is to discover new scents. Or, I will try a couple of drops on my skin, and experience how they warm up on me over time. I don't think you should rush into selecting a fragrance; the first "hit" is fleeting, but it's the middle and bass notes that you'll live with, and they take time to fully blossom.

When I was seventeen and training in a ballet company, I learned a trick from one of the older dancers, a beautiful, sophisticated French girl whom I adored and admired. She sprayed fragrance onto her hands. "Then," she told me in her delicious French accent, "when I shake the hand of a man, upon noticing it later he asks himself, 'Now who smelled so wonderful?'" In fact, there are lots of surprising places you can wear perfume—don't just dab it behind your ears! And remember: Perfume makes you beautiful in the dark.

SCENTED DRAWER LINERS It's great to line your lingerie drawer with fragrant paper. My friend Barbara brought back a lot of inexpensive little lavender-filled bags from her trip to Provence. I got hooked on having sweetly scented underclothes, so now lavender sachets are a must for me. If you grow lavender, you can make your own. One critical fragrance "don't," however; try to steer clear of mothballs. To me they smell of death and decay and are particularly aging if the odor is still clinging to your clothes when you step out. Instead, try cedarwood blocks, which smell wonderfully woodsy and are almost as effective.

THE POWER OF AROMATHERAPY Aromatherapy is the art of using essential oils extracted from aromatic plants to enhance beauty and health. Apart from the physical benefits to the body, the essences have subtle effects on the mind and emotions. (Virgin Atlantic offers aromatherapy massages to de-stress their upper-class travelers—and to help combat jet lag!) I love to incorporate aromatherapy essential oils—distilled from herbs and spices, woods, flowers, and resins—into massages and baths. You can also vaporize them with hot water or burn them in a special aromatherapy burner, which you can find in specialty shops like The Body Shop, department stores, and even some grocery stores.

ESSENTIAL ESSENTIAL OILS Some of the most popular (and powerful) essential oils and their claims to fame include:

- BASIL: This essential oil has been used for thousands of years to treat chest problems and digestive problems; this refreshing oil clears the head and brings strength and clarity to the mind.
- CLARY SAGE: This warm, nutty scent has a euphoric quality, uplifting the spirits when feelings are low, promoting well-being and relaxation.
- GERANIUM: It has an antiseptic effect and is stimulating to the senses. It can help relieve premenstrual tension and promote hormonal balance and is now being used for menopause problems. It also helps to speed up the lymphatic system.
- JASMINE: This is extremely expensive, as vast quantities of flowers are needed to extract even a tiny amount of oil. Most often used for "women's problems," such as menstrual cramps, jasmine is also known as an aphrodisiac and antidepressant and is supposed to impart confidence.
- LAVENDER: The most versatile essential oil: a painkiller, antidepressant, insect repellant, and decongestant. Lavender is also used to restore a state of balance in the mind and body. (It's good for inducing sleep, too; I like to put a couple of drops on my pillow or on my sleep mask.)
- MELISSA: This strongly lemon-scented oil is soothing both to body and mind. Its overall effect is a gentle, but effective, tonic. Paracelsus called it the "elixir of life"!
- NEROLI: From the flowers of the bitter orange, this is often used as an aphrodisiac. It can reduce depression and anxiety, stimulate the growth of healthy new skin cells, and reduce muscle spasms.
- PEPPERMINT: A widely used oil for digestive upsets, stomach pain, colds, and flu, it's also said to aid clear thinking. A cold compress of peppermint can help to relieve migraine and headaches.
- ROSE: Rose is known as the "queen of essential oils." This expensive oil has a powerful effect on the circulation, digestive, and nervous systems. It's long been used as an aphrodisiac. (The Romans used to scatter rose petals on the bridal bed . . .)
- ROSEMARY: This was one of the first plants used in medicine; it has a stimulating effect on the brain and nervous system and clears the mind. Described as the "middle-age executive's best friend," for its use as a tonic for the heart, liver, and gall bladder and to help lower blood cholesterol levels.

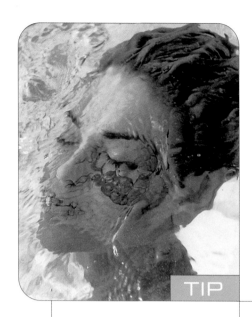

TIP

BATH TIME BLISS
Aromatherapy oils are powerful mood-shifters. As you discover more about the oils, you'll learn how to use them to achieve a particular frame of mind. In the meantime, however, here are a few essential oil blends, for different purposes:

TO UNWIND:
4 drops cypress,
2 drops lavender,
2 drops cajuput

AS AN APHRODISIAC:
4 drops patchouli,
4 drops ylang-ylang,
2 drops jasmine

FOR INSTANT
GET-UP-AND-GO:
4 drops tangerine,
4 drops bergamot

WHEN YOU'RE
FEELING LOW:
4 drops lemon,
4 drops ylang-ylang

AS A WINTER IMMUNE
SYSTEM BOOSTER:
4 drops tea tree,
2 drops eucalpytus,
2 drops lavender

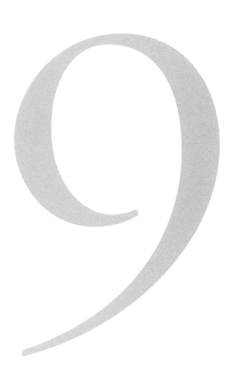

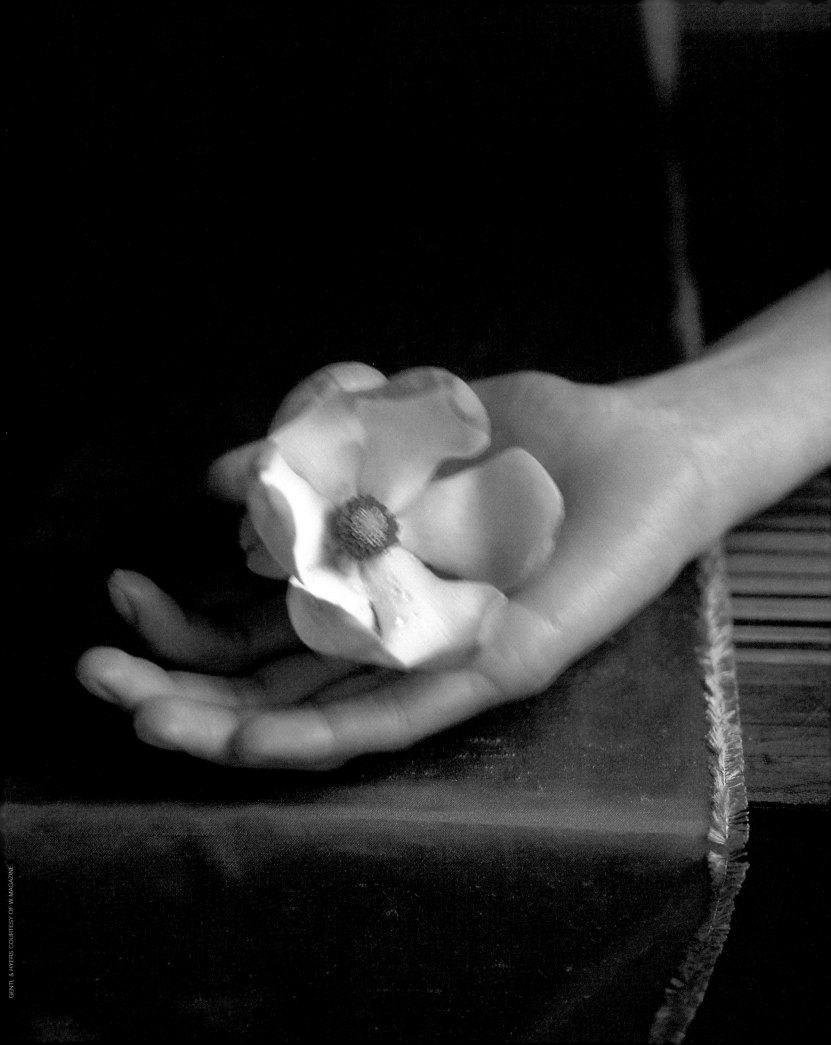

LIFE:
THE GREAT BALANCING ACT

Our twenties were a time of searching and building; we ricocheted through life, often fueled by the expectations of others, trying to "find ourselves," combined, of course, with a complete naiveté about the world and its meaning. Then our thirties whizzed by as we fulfilled our duties or chased our ambitions with single-minded drive and determination. Now that we are in or approaching midlife, we are in the perfect position to ask ourselves, "What's next?"

Midlife is right in the middle. The perfect place to find balance. We can see where we have been and where we are going. We have enough experiences behind us now that we can measure and manage situations better—evaluate the importance of certain relationships, decide where and how we want to spend our time. Midlife is the point when we must realize, "Whoa, this is my life, my movie—how do I want to spend the rest of it?" It is time to establish our own blueprint for the future. The first step is searching for (or maintaining) our balance.

Perhaps you've reached a point where your responsibilities seem to be in order, your children have left home or they don't need as much of your time and energy. Although this newfound time may feel a bit strange, overwhelming, even scary, it can actually mark a new beginning. After all, time is the one thing that can allow us to discover possibilities, so we should cherish, celebrate, and take advantage of this gift—enjoying the new freedom and opportunity more time and more energy afford us. It can be difficult for someone who has always put other people first, to feel comfortable with this focus on themselves. It's simple: If you don't take care of yourself, you can't take care of others. Who nurtures the nurturer?

A life that's too focused on one area—work, responsibilities, a relationship, external goals—is most likely out of balance, incomplete, and potentially unstable. Think of a tree: when a tree grows, it sends out all of its energy to form many branches. The tree can risk losing a branch or two, because it has many others that will help retain its shape and form. But if the tree puts out only one branch, and sends all its energy to that one limb, then it would be vulnerable to any of the stresses nature sent its way. Any storm, wind, or snow would put too much pressure on the single limb—probably causing it to snap under the added weight, or even topple the tree itself.

We, too, must develop other branches—interests that strengthen and nourish us, especially during times of challenge and stress. So it's time to develop the other parts of ourselves that may have been neglected. This is exciting! It's almost like a new life, a second chance, with new beginnings and fresh opportunities. We can grow in different ways than we did in our twenties—because we have experience and the wisdom, strength, and perspective of time. In the flush of youth, maybe you wanted to become a movie star, be elected president, write a best-seller, or marry a prince . . . living happily ever after, of course. Maybe, at times, you felt disappointed by your reality.

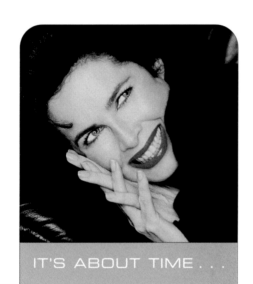

IT'S ABOUT TIME . . .

. . .to decide how we want to spend the rest of our lives. To get rid of the excess baggage, heal our lives—and find balance, making time for ourselves and others so that we can make the most of the next twenty, thirty, forty years of life's adventure. Living better—maybe even living longer—is all a question of attitude. Life isn't always easy. But we develop our own personal philosophies that enable us to survive hardships—and experience the joy of celebrating victories. So let me share with you my insights.

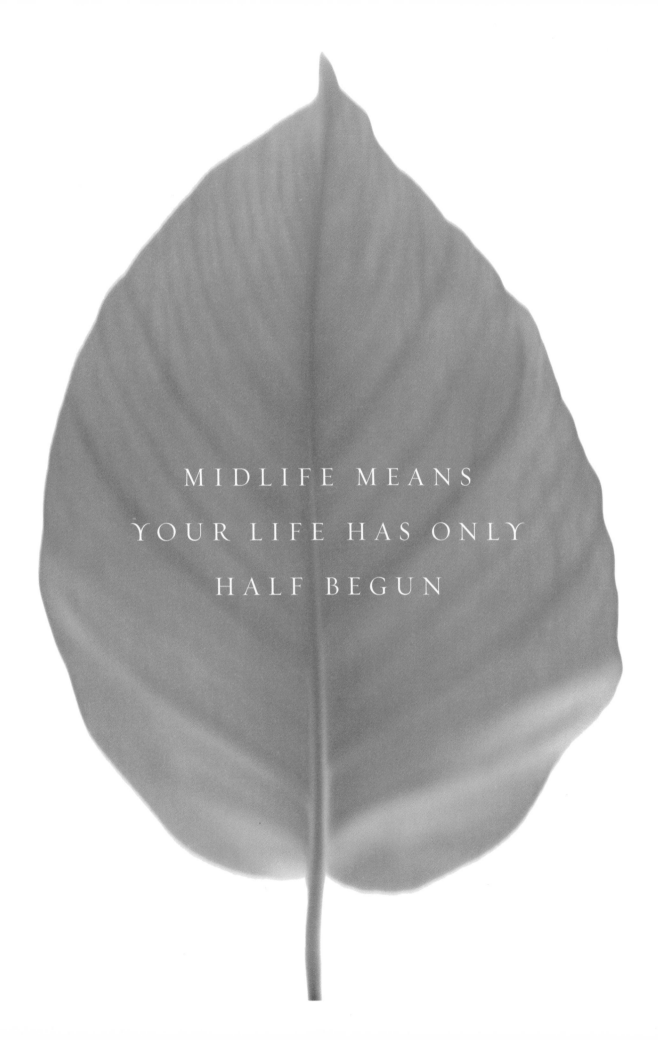

MIDLIFE MEANS
YOUR LIFE HAS ONLY
HALF BEGUN

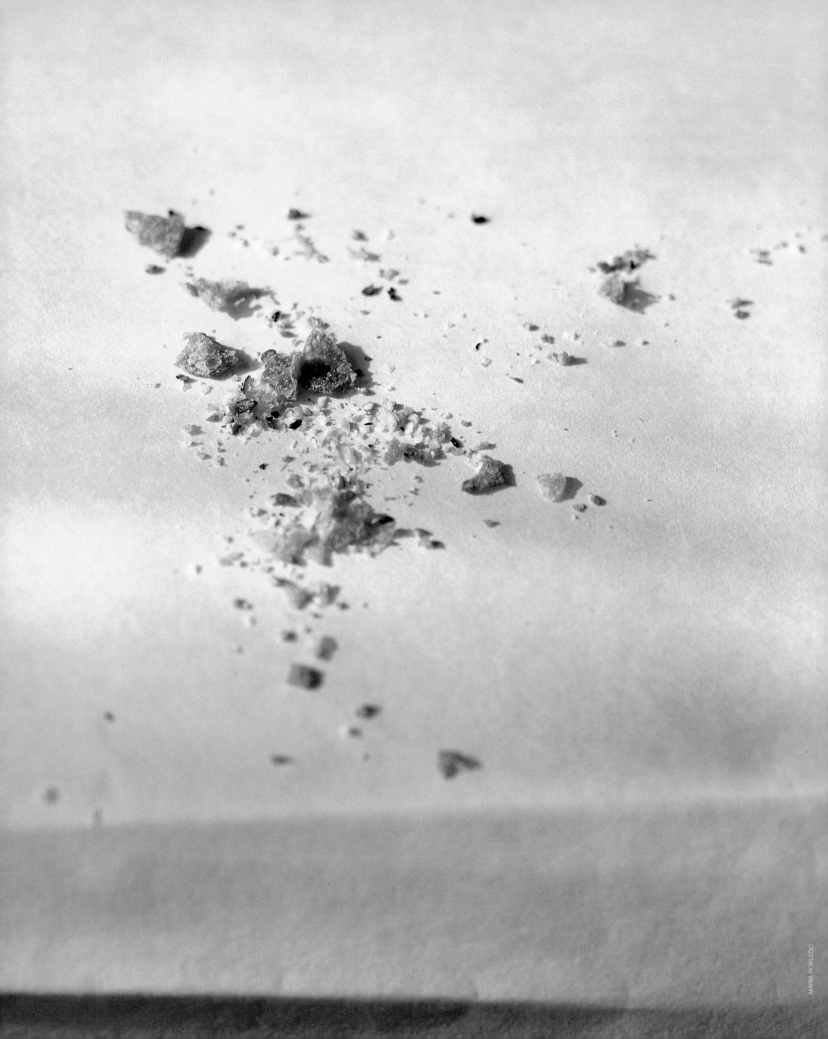

With midlife—thank heavens—comes a more realistic outlook. By forty, we should all know what our needs are and have an inkling about how to fulfill them—pacing ourselves, sensing when our batteries are running down, and recharging them before they do. Managing the pace and content of our life is a vital part of balance and it comes from doing the things that support us on a regular basis. It's not about, "I must lose six pounds before a vacation"; it's about establishing a healthy eating lifestyle. It's not about walking seven miles one day and then crashing as a couch potato for the next six. It's about an active lifestyle that incorporates exercise into each day, every day.

Losing someone was a tremendous reminder to me of the fragility of life. It made me grateful for what I have. I often think about something my friend Diane, who is a well-known therapist, told me. Her husband had a terrible habit of leaving crumbs all over every time he used the kitchen. She was grumbling about having to clean up after him when a powerful revelation hit her: If her husband weren't there, there wouldn't be a crumbly mess. Her entire attitude dramatically changed right there and then, because the very existence of those crumbs meant that he existed, and she was so very grateful that he did. (I wouldn't say she's now grateful for the crumbs, but it made her feel a whole lot better about them.)

Gratitude is an incredible balancer. We all have moments when we are down or, in certain circumstances, even feel victimized. I find it helps if I write down what I am grateful for. Sometimes, I am surprised by how long the list is. When something is taken away, that's often when you realize how much you value what you had. Don't wait until then. There is so much that we take for granted, including the ability to walk, breathe, see, hear, and smell: Just imagine life without these gifts.

Rather than wish your life away, always thinking about what could have or should have been . . . longing for yesterday or dreaming about an unrealistic future, try to Be Here Now. Don't miss out on the present.

Another secret of balance is to be flexible—not to have life so "worked out" that the slightest change of plan throws you into a dither or have so rigid a life that it ceases to be an adventure. You have to grant each day its own personality. Computers crash, kids get sick, cars break down—and you have to let it go. It happens . . . and it's called Life. At this stage, you probably have the perspective to laugh some of it off. Try asking yourself, "Will I be worrying about this on my deathbed?" If not, let it go.

Midlife is the time to make sense of the deeper things, to develop a personal philosophy about this adventure we are sharing called Life so that we can play our individual role most effectively. It's about time to feel more relaxed, to laugh at ourselves more, to be more generous. There is no point in trying to change the world without changing ourselves, first. This will have the most impact.

Review the things you want to improve about yourself and start making those shifts. I truly believe that if you follow some of the suggestions in this book—even the simplest ideas, from de-junking your wardrobe or boosting your energy to living with fragrance or learning to meditate—you will find a wonderful new clarity that enables you to tune into your own instincts and insights about life, people, the future. And to find your balance, the secret of true beauty.

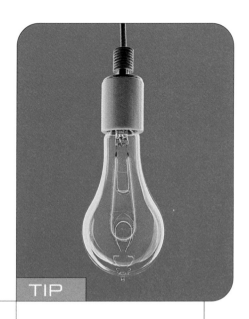

I first recognized that I desperately needed organization in my life after the loss of my husband and the destruction of my home. The turning point for me came with the need to repair my house. The severity of the situation gave me the urgency to change. I had come to the point where I could no longer be a disorganized, inefficient person. It was one of those moments in life when the lightbulb finally goes on. I realized the way I had been was not going to support who I wanted and needed to be.

And as I started to learn the skills (and joys) of organization, I felt literally empowered. I discovered a sense of freedom, felt focused, and became less stressed each day as, step by step, I slowly regained control and order over my life.

IT'S ABOUT MORE TIME Time is one of the greatest luxuries of all; the one thing no woman can ever have enough of. Leaving behind the intense drive and overwhelming responsibilities of our twenties and thirties can be liberating. But ask any woman at midlife to describe the greatest gift she could imagine and she will still probably answer, "more time."

One of the best ways to give yourself more time, every single day, is to become better organized. It's about not spending fifteen minutes searching for your car keys, ten minutes trying to locate a phone number, thirty minutes correcting a billing mess because you mailed the check three days late.

There is so much that we can't control in life. But we can control our closets, our desks, our space. Buy a Sharp electronic organizer, de-junk every season, find the perfect laundry sorter. Added up, these organizational secrets can shave hours from your schedule, giving you the gift of more time for yourself—to read a book, take a walk, or spend time with your family.

HEALING
YOUR LIFE

Healing yourself has to do with being "whole." By midlife, we are usually carrying around a fair amount of excess emotional baggage—and it's we who suffer. We have to decide whether we want to lug around this extra baggage for the rest of our lives. So many conversations I have with women have to do with old, old issues they still have with ex-husbands, mothers, fathers, children. Midlife is the moment to heal your relationships, unpack the suitcase, and put out the trash.

What you think about triggers how you feel. So if you carry around angry, bitter thoughts and memories, you will feel angry and bitter. By this point in life, it's important to ask: How much more time do we want to spend with such negative feelings? Now is the time to heal, as best we can. Easier said than done? If a past relationship or difficult past event is still affecting my life, I find it's helpful to go within and address what happened and what was felt. Ask yourself: "How do I feel about it?" Then acknowledge that feeling and let it go.

I believe that it's crucial to have everything out in the open. There will always be plenty of things that bother you in a relationship, but if you keep the lines of communication open, saying what you feel, you have the chance to develop a much deeper emotional connection. It can be tricky: You have to find ways to say things that won't hurt people or send them flying off the handle. But there are ways to sit somebody down and say: "I need you to know how I feel." This approach gives the other person the space to consider what's going on in your universe. It is communicating your needs. It doesn't necessarily blame the other person for how you feel or place them in the wrong. The flip side is that on an ongoing basis you have to be able to listen and try to understand the other person's feelings as well. Consideration and respect can then form the basis of your relationships.

Heal your relationships now so that you don't have regrets later. One of the most painful things that can happen in our lives is to lose someone and have things left unsaid. There are several ways to deal with this.

I have talked with therapists in clinics like Sierra Tucson and The Meadows, who shared this simple and helpful technique: Sit down, put a chair opposite you, several feet away. Imagine the person you want to speak to sitting there facing you, say out loud the things you want to say—things that you may never have been able to say in real life to that invisible person. This can be very helpful to release pent-up feelings that may be harmful to you in the long run.

You may want to call the person you've had an argument or falling out with, although phone confrontation can be difficult. If possible, it's better to do it in person. (A phone being slammed down can be a blow to the heart!) If this is too extreme or difficult, try writing a letter. The phrasing of a letter is obviously very important. My friend Diane, who has published many books on the subject, suggests starting with the phrase, "I need your help." If he or she cannot see you at that moment, ask when would be a good time to discuss things, then follow up and make sure it happens. When you meet, simply say: "These are the things I need to tell you, that I am having a problem with." Posing it as your problem makes it infinitely less threatening for the other person. Never attack or blame. If you corner even the tiniest animal, it will fight back, and people are the same way.

If you really need help shifting emotional baggage, try therapy. I think that, if you can afford it, therapy can be extremely helpful. It can be very insightful to hold up a mirror to your life and gain new understanding. There are many, many kinds of therapy and I have included a list of some of the books that I have found helpful (see suggested reading list). For more involved problems, you should ask friends or your family doctor for a therapist recommendation (see Resources).

Maybe you're carrying a lot of envy, anger, and jealousy. These are among what Eastern philosophers call the "inner enemies": anger, jealousy, envy, delusion, desire, pride, and laziness. They are things we all feel at times, that we must work to overcome. They are negative emotions that prevent us from achieving our potential—that don't allow us to feel happy.

It's important to watch for the "inner enemies." When an emotion like envy or pride appears, we can spot it quickly and be aware of how it makes us feel less than we truly are. I find that by identifying and observing it, the negativity loses its power and hold over us.

It's simply a question of understanding how we might be undermining ourselves as we go through life. Most of us have negative tapes that continuously play in our head. So if you have a tape that brings you down, eject it immediately—and exchange it for a more positive one. Transformation can be surprisingly easy, if you stay alert and work at it a bit. If you want to be a loving, generous person, you must be loving and generous to yourself first.

Another important part of healing is to reward yourself when you do well. If nobody is there to tell you how great you are, stand in the middle of the room and congratulate yourself: "I did a great job today!" Make the effort to applaud

TIP

Write every negative sentiment you feel in a letter. Put it in an envelope and burn it. Fire is an incredible cleanser. Do it in a ceremonial way, stating: "I give this up"—especially if the person is no longer there or you can't speak to them.

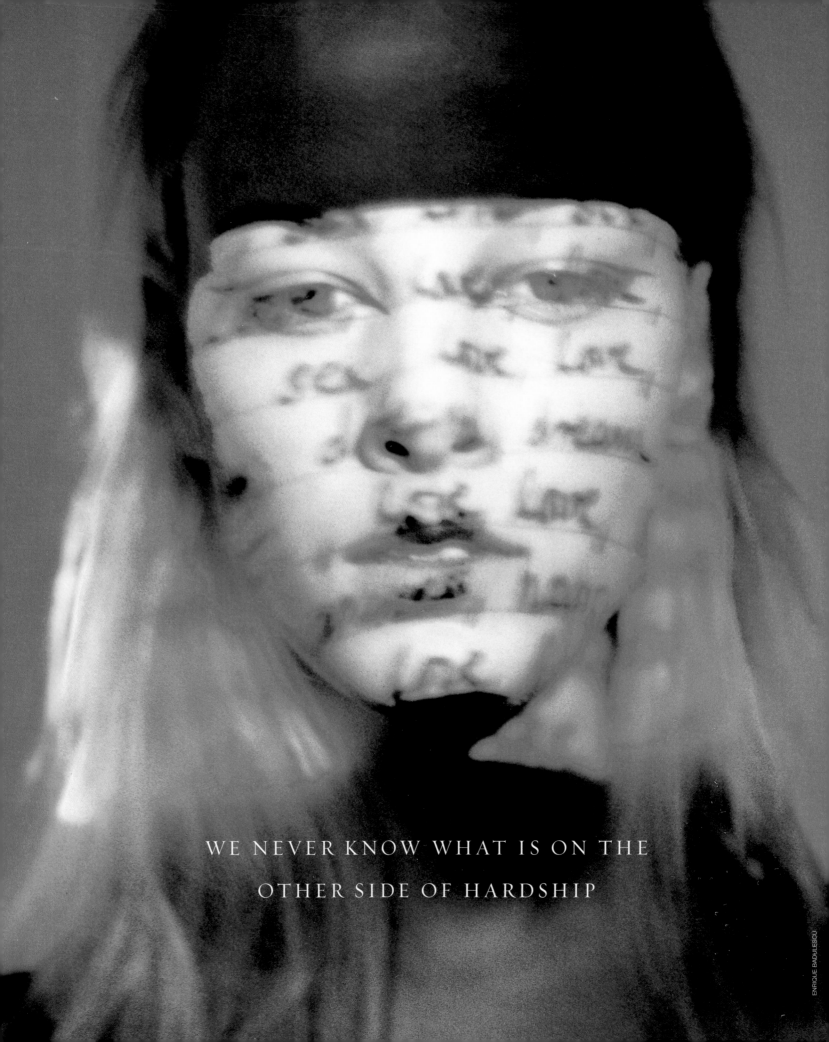

WE NEVER KNOW WHAT IS ON THE
OTHER SIDE OF HARDSHIP

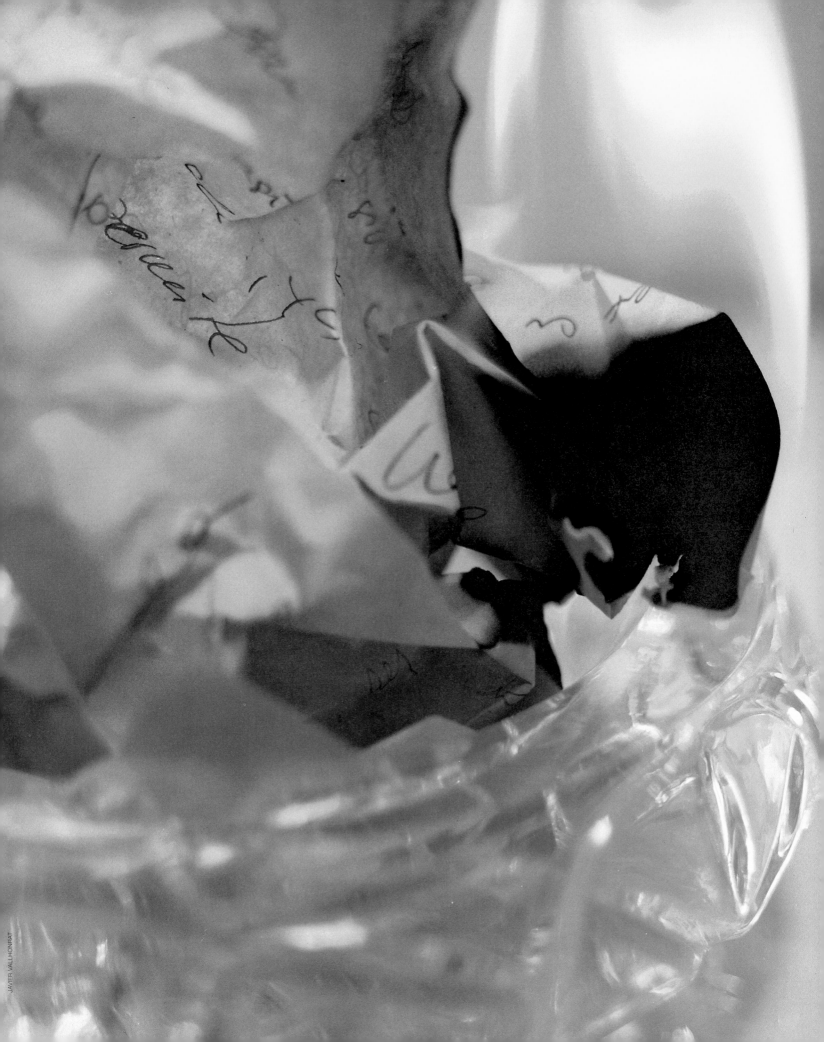

others as well. When people are encouraged and acknowledged, what they can achieve is almost limitless. People perform better when they hear they did well. It's human nature.

Don't assume that anyone is psychic: State your needs. If you need a hug, say "I need a hug!" It is healthy to recognize and communicate your needs. It's also important to have healthy boundaries, to let others know what you—as a parent, a lover, a professional, a friend—will and won't accept. This makes it easier to avoid rifts.

Part of healing our lives depends on relinquishing the past. This might mean letting go of a younger you—the you that may have been center stage once upon a time—and learning to appreciate the new you.

I like to think the body I have is a vehicle that gets me through life. Therefore, I take care of it. I feed and exercise it, rest it, and keep it clean. I am more than a body, however, more than a model, a chick, a babe, a dame, a broad, or any of the other labels stuck on women. None of these labels fully defines us—and some clearly diminish us. In our forties, we must define who this new woman is and who we are to become. We also need to step aside and gracefully allow other younger people to share center stage. It is the moment in life for us to move to our new, and I feel, more important, more valuable, more exciting place in time. Outside the spotlight of youth, we will all find something much more interesting and fulfilling.

Instead of focusing on what we've lost, we can focus on what we've gained over the years: intelligence, wisdom, experience and humor, among other things, and the daring to share them all. Let's face it—we're all going to get a wrinkle or three. But for me, it's all worth it, because of what I've earned and learned en route. Life is an adventure, and it doesn't have just one peak. It can have many . . . and only if you stop staring back regretfully over your shoulder can you see the wonderful panorama ahead.

YOUR SPACE
THE FINAL FRONTIER

You have to feel that somewhere, you have a place of your own. Everyone needs a place—even if it's just a corner in their house—to call their own; an area that can act as a source of sanity. If all else fails, you can return to your space and shut out the demands of the world, even for a moment. You can retreat there as often as you need to recharge yourself. Virginia Woolf said that every woman needs a room of her own, but with families and partners, that's often an impossible dream.

I met with a woman not long ago who was having a really hard time: She was in a state of exhaustion and near collapse. She had nurtured and given everything she had to her family and had absolutely nothing left for herself. While telling me her story, she realized that everyone had their own place in the house except her. Even the dog had its own space! So I suggested that she find some small space of her own within her home. She loved the concept and became more and more excited about it the more she considered the possibilities. She even insisted on driving me home to show me where "her space" could be. She realized that she could transform a useless storage area into an incredibly special place where she could withdraw, closing the door on the world when she needed to. A place that would nurture, protect, and transform her.

My husband died and I had to move and start over; I needed to create a place that was a haven to come home to, a place that would support and nurture me through this difficult time. I spent a lot of time and care on this space because I knew it would give so much back to me. It's a small apartment, but it's filled with light and warmth and with objects I treasure—special things I have discovered in antique markets. I took a lot of effort to make my space wonderful for me. I used soft colors, made sure I always had flowers, hung transparent curtains that let light in, and filled the space with music and candles. I wanted to achieve a sense of airiness and peace because I knew it would nourish me and keep me from feeling empty inside.

JUST SAY NO
SHEDDING BAD HABITS

At this stage in your life, part of the process of deciding who you are and who you're going to be is realizing what needs to be eliminated, what doesn't work for you anymore. It's also about recognizing what in your life is habitual. Because chances are good that, when something is habitual, it is controlling you.

Step one is observing yourself. At midlife, you want to take the time to find out: Who is this person that has come this far? What are the things you do repeatedly? If they are positive habits that support the woman you want to be, then great: if you're regularly exercising, then for heaven's sake, leave it alone! But you may have habits that don't support the emerging you. Take an inventory; literally get a pencil and paper and write them down as they come to you. Do you drink too much? Smoke? Take too many over-the-counter painkillers? Just because a drug is prescribed, or you can buy it in a pharmacy, doesn't mean you can't develop a dependency. If you do not know where to start, then ask someone you trust: Are there some things I could change? (Be careful of the people who say, "Don't change a thing!") You usually know! Maybe you're not good at disciplining yourself to get up early or not getting enough regular exercise or your eating habits could be improved. A bad habit doesn't have to be a vice.

So review, contemplate, try to recognize the negative habits that can hold you back from being the most you can be. Very often, bad habits fill a hole in your life. The practices elsewhere in this book should help to fill this void so that you don't need a crutch: walking, exercise, and meditation, in particular, will help.

But let's be realistic: overcoming bad habits can still be difficult. Bad habits are usually acquired over years. We may gossip too much, smoke constantly, watch TV mindlessly, bicker with our partner over nothing—and we may

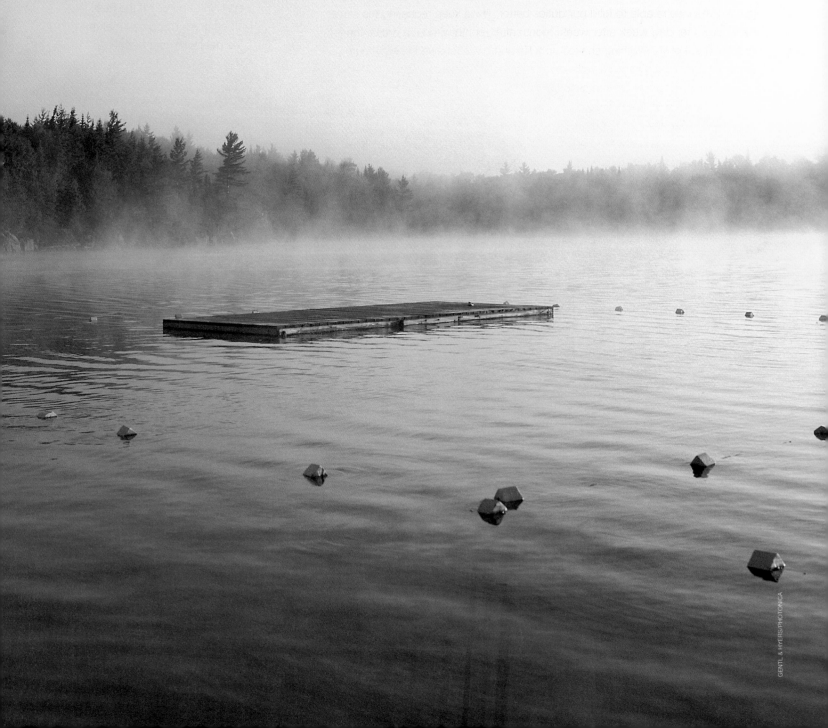

"NOBODY HAS EVER SAID ON HER DEATH BED,

'I WISH I'D SPENT MORE TIME IN THE OFFICE'"

MARY JO WEAVER

have been doing it for decades. Another immensely bad habit is to put ourselves down constantly, undermining ourselves and our progress. But bad habits can be broken. The recognition and acknowledgment of them is the first positive step. We all have them. Join the club.

GETTING AWAY

The point of getting away is to come back with more to offer. We should take care to replenish ourselves before we're so empty that it becomes an emergency. Then we're able to fulfill our duties better. If we keep repeating the same cycle, day after day, week after week, month after month without a break, the joy is drained out of life. Nothing shakes up a life and gives renewed energy more than a change of scenery. It's refreshing, and everyone needs to be refreshed.

Taking a break often makes us feel guilty, though; colleagues and family sometimes make us feel we are being selfish for taking time for ourselves. We have to get over any guilt about putting ourselves at the top of the list for a change. Learn to find a way to acknowledge, this is okay for me; I give myself permission to get away.

In reality, many therapists and counselors maintain taking time for yourself actually communicates to others that you have value—and if you have value, then they have value. If you don't take care of yourself, for example, what that can communicate to a child—whose life is so intrinsically entwined with yours—is that you are not worth the effort. If you're not worth it, in modeling themselves after you, they will learn to think that they aren't worth it either. If you don't set an example of caring for yourself, they will probably repeat the same pattern. By taking some time out, you're conveying that you have the strength of character, the intelligence, and the responsibility to take care of your personal needs. And is that selfish?

So listen to the alarm bells and take action before you've run out of energy. Avoid overloading your schedule. Pace yourself—so that somebody else doesn't have to pick you up off the floor.

For me, February is the trickiest month. I tend not to take summer vacations, so by the end of February, I can't take much more. Nowadays, that's when I schedule my break; if I stretch myself through to March without one, it's me that breaks. Most of us can extend our workload if we try, but we have to take time to smell the roses. (So schedule mini-breaks, too: try to get away each day from your duties for just a moment to be in Nature—gaze at the moon, the autumn leaves, the sunset, or the stars—and escape momentarily.)

Don't just think of getting away as something you need to do on your own. For relationships, it is essential to spend time together as a couple, away from the children (or parents that you may be caring for).

My friend Christine, who has three children under five, realized her mar-

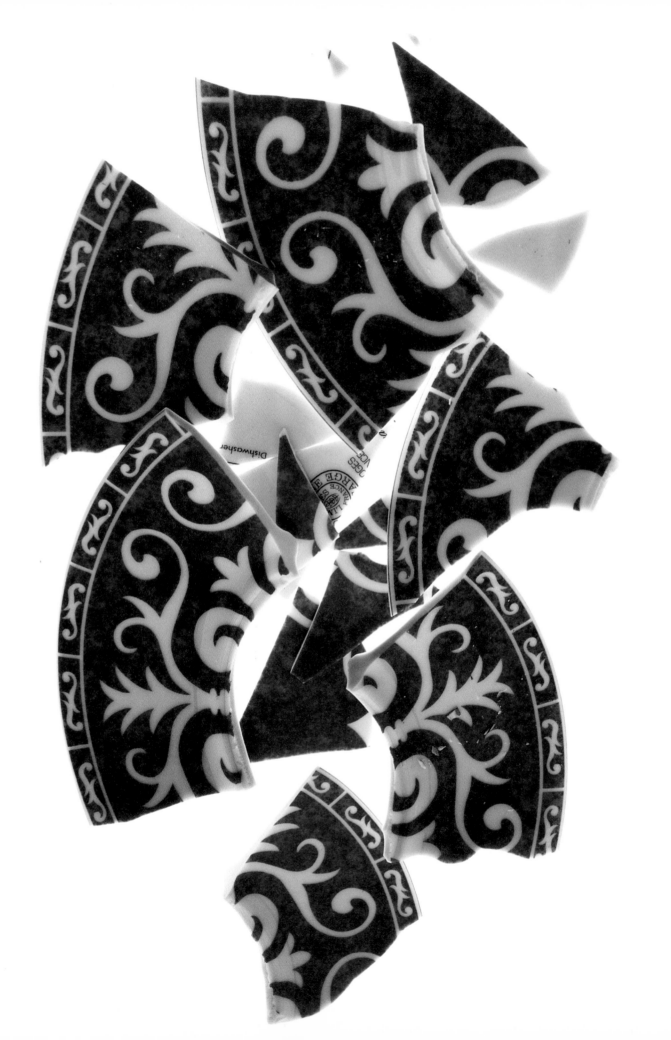

riage was not getting the attention it deserved. All of their energy was being spent on the demands of their children and there was nothing left for the two of them. Instead of obsessing or complaining about the situation, Christine took action: she booked an inexpensive five-day cruise to Alaska—just for the two of them. Her husband is a high-powered executive who has difficulty taking time off, she is a mother of three who doesn't usually have a moment to spare. But somehow they managed, and it turned their marriage around, heading disaster off at the pass. They still find it hard to get away for long periods of time, but now they've made a pact: for birthdays and anniversaries, they take turns planning a surprise for each other and this is their time. It becomes highly creative; they might pack a picnic lunch and drive to Sonoma—each time it's different. It gives them something in their lives that is not a) about work and b) about the kids . . . and is so rejuvenating for them and their relationship.

So be inspired. Send away for brochures; tear out articles from magazines that feed your dreams of "The Great Escape." Whether you go alone, with a friend, or with everyone—from great-grandma to your second-cousin-twice-removed—just do it . . .

SURVIVING HARDSHIPS

We are not in control of most of the larger events in our lives, but we can control our attitude toward them. Personally, I have arrived at the realization that the greater the problem, the greater the possibility of transformation. The philosopher Sir Laurens van der Post, who I admire immensely, wrote that "the problems of life, the problems of the universe, the problems with man are our most precious possessions because they are the raw materials of our redemption." So, no problem, no redemption. I try to keep that thought tucked away; it doesn't make an incident any less painful, but I have faith I will eventually discover the lesson that life was trying to teach me.

As a friend once explained to me, life is not flat land and easy coasting; it's hills and mountains (and only sometimes do we get to coast down them!). You have to be prepared and ready; then when you get to the mountains, you are better equipped to climb them. By nurturing yourself, by taking time to go into Nature, by being a loving, kind person and searching for the true values in your life, you will be better equipped to deal with hardships as they come. Caring for yourself physically also helps you to face difficulties: You achieve an inner balance as well as a stronger body. Then the emotional bank is a credit line and you can draw on it. One of my favorite sayings is that grace and self-effort are two wings of the bird. It really is the day-to-day, regular work you do on yourself that becomes a source of strength during hardships.

The most difficult hardship we can face in life is the loss of people we love: friends, partners, parents, and children. Another of Sir Laurens's observa-

Usually, a destructive habit goes hand-in-hand with denial. So if someone suggests to you that you have a problem, pay attention; if it's significant enough for them to bring it to your attention, there may very well be something in what they're saying. If I hear something once about myself, I can dismiss it; if I hear it twice, then to me it's worth looking at. If you want to become a new person, this is part of the tallying up: What are other people saying that I can act upon? Review regularly. When you conquer a bad habit, suddenly you have a different view on life; you're standing in another place. The vista has changed and perhaps you can see more clearly other areas of your life that you could work on. Reviewing is creative. You're living consciously. Remember, the obstacles are there to make life interesting; they ground you. Any problem is a challenge for you to become more.

tions is that we live in a society in which the idea of death does not exist. It's true; we brush aside the thought of death; and therefore it's such a shock when it arrives. But by contemplating death and confronting our own mortality, we have the possibility to get more out of life. People with a life-threatening illness so often say that having looked death in the face, they appreciate every single day, every moment, so much more intensely.

Society teaches us that problems are bad, even shameful. If we're having difficulties, it must mean we are doing something wrong. So we may blame ourselves or feel victimized: "Why me? Why is this happening to me?" In the course of life, we inevitably encounter incredibly painful situations: bereavement, job loss, fires, and financial catastrophes. These crises can act as the tools that we use to get to know ourselves—and to grow. We often do not know who we are until tragedy strikes. Then we are forced to go deeper within, accessing strengths we may never know we had.

Change is painful; most people don't want to change; few people like what is unfamiliar. Sometimes it takes a disaster or an upheaval to pry us out of the habitual way we live and take us to the next level. When a dramatic event shakes the foundations of our life—divorce, loss of money or a job, a death in the family—it is terrifying and painful. But I try to remind myself that we are not given more than we can handle. By taking it one day at a time, eventually you may find an even better job, there might be a new person that is more loving out there, or you may discover new, hidden talents, as I did.

Life, for some reason that we can't understand yet, is asking more of us, and that is what we have to remember. Agree to embark on the adventure of finding out what that could be. Life was asking me to become a different person. As a result of my loss, I went on to develop my own company, write a book, become a businesswoman, and find the passion for what I believe in. This evolution gives me a happiness that in the dark days of the past I simply could not have imagined for myself.

Dealing with grief is very individual, but it's very, very unhealthy to avoid addressing it. The emotions will be released in some other form—probably as illness. The suppressed grief might emerge as bitterness, frustration, or victimization. Therefore, it is very important to confront your grief—probably sooner, rather than later—before it has a chance to do you more harm.

Connecting with a therapist, a group, or a support network can be very helpful for many people. Talk, talk, and talk with a friend that knows you. You should never feel shy about picking up the phone when you are in need. It can also make someone else feel wanted and needed. It takes courage to make the move and can leave you vulnerable, but other people usually understand how hard it is to reach out—and knowing that, they will usually be there for you when you do.

But be reassured: Grief does run its course. We may never forget the person we have lost. We should never forget that person, but grief does finds its place over time.

We never know what is on the other side of hardship. We never know what treasures we may find. For me, my loss presented me with the chance for total transformation. After a time, the experience left me with so many things: more compassion, more understanding, more humor, and much more love. It made me become selective about how I wanted to spend my time and with whom. My whole life has changed, on so many levels. I believe I am a better person with even more capacity for happiness, because of what I went through. Even if it doesn't feel that way at the time, opportunity, disguised as misfortune, can bring about changes in us that are so dramatic, we may not even recognize the old person we were.

Trust that it is so.

CELBRATING VICTORIES

There are little ones and there are big ones and you've got to celebrate them all. Every day is a victory! So when you get through the day doing the best you can do, acknowledge your success. Life's ups and downs never end; we have the good times and the bad times throughout our lives. By honoring the victories, we help restore ourselves, and are ready for the more difficult times around the bend. Certainly, when hardships end, as they eventually do, we have to celebrate those moments too.

We shouldn't wait for someone else to recognize and applaud our triumphs. After all, when was the last time someone applauded your clean laundry, cried, "Bravo!" for that great meal, or thanked you for staying late to meet a deadline. Congratulate yourself. Say your own "Bravo." Connect, share a victory with a friend.

Birthdays are victories. Forty, fifty, that's a victory! Don't shrink away from them. A girlfriend of mine insisted that there was absolutely no way she was going to celebrate her fiftieth birthday. When I pointed out to her that turning fifty was better than the alternative, she had to admit that on that note, fifty looked pretty good.

When my nephew, Duran, turned thirteen, my sister Darilyn wanted to make a very special birthday celebration. She strung several rows of ribbon across the kitchen, with photographs of his life from birth; then handed him a pair of scissors. Carefully he cut through each ribbon that recorded his life, one by one, as his family cheered him on. Celebrated in this unique way, Duran's transition from childhood to his teens was something the whole family could share.

Once upon a time, we acknowledged a girl's journey into womanhood with a celebration. In Naomi Wolfe's book *Promiscuities*, she writes in depth about the lack of ceremony or acknowledgment of our transition from girlhood to womanhood, and the negative effects this can have on women today. She writes of how certain Indian tribes, at one time, would row a young girl who had reached puberty out into the middle of a lake. The young girl then had to swim back to shore while the entire village waited to welcome her. She was then recognized by her tribe as a woman. (Of course, most teenage girls today would rather die than have their first period celebrated, but it does go to show how much of the magical ritual we have lost in our lives.)

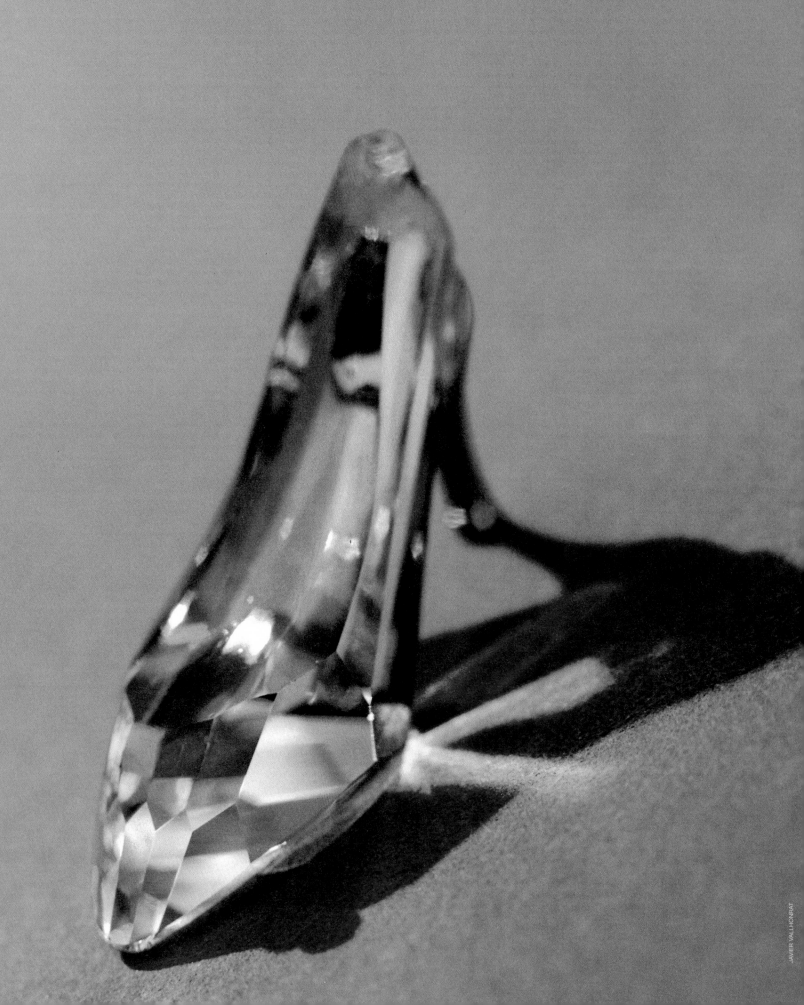

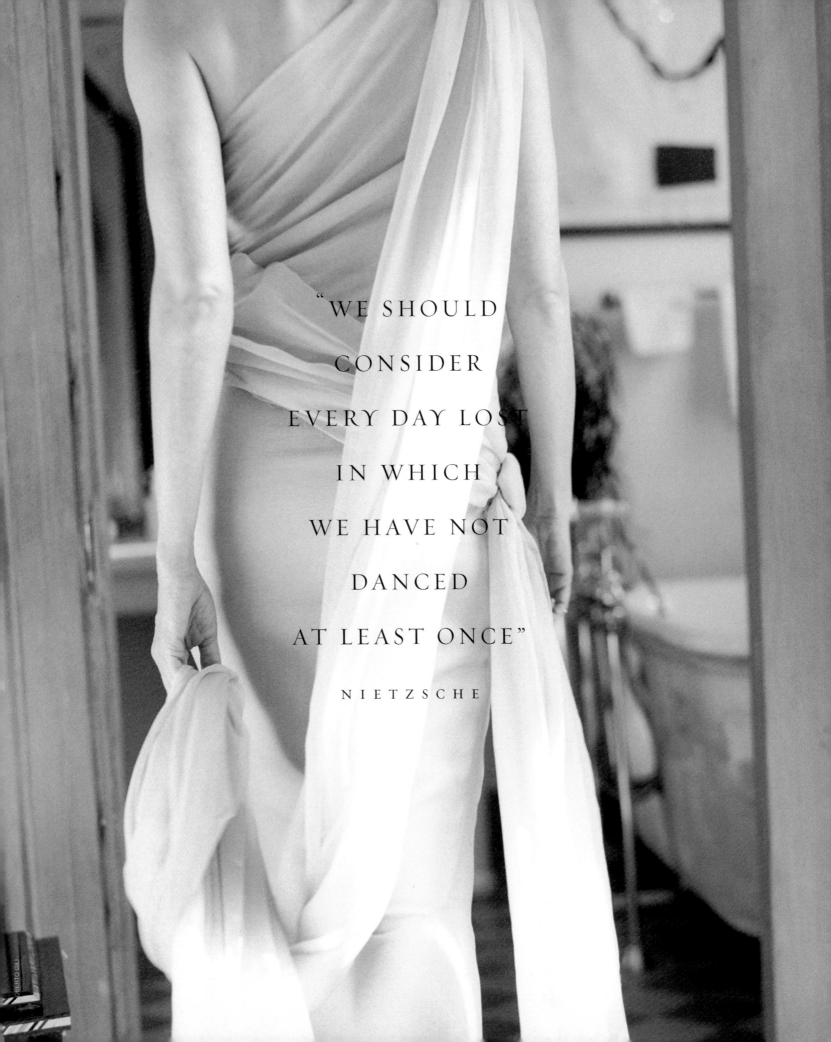

"WE SHOULD
CONSIDER
EVERY DAY LOST
IN WHICH
WE HAVE NOT
DANCED
AT LEAST ONCE"

NIETZSCHE

I try to make a point, however, to acknowledge all of the victories, large and small, in my life. Before I go to sleep, I like to review the day saying, "That was good . . . this was great." I find that the feeling of gratitude enhances what I already have. I will often make a list of what I am grateful for: being thankful for the day, for the sunshine, for the smile that so-and-so gave me. It is about finding the little gems in life that we can string together to make something truly beautiful.

Going down a dress size is a victory worth celebrating. The first time you walk three miles is a victory. Finishing any project is a victory. Getting through a day when it felt like you were swimming through molasses is a victory. So congratulate yourself.

DREAMS & GOALS

There is no question, life would be dull without dreams. Dreams are what get your motor going, excite you, start you thinking about all the possibilities in life. You need time to dream of what might be possible. This kind of dreaming isn't escapism; it's another form of creative visualization that can help us get there from here. And we all need a secret place inside us where we can cultivate the magic of life.

Out of dreams grow goals. Our dreams provide us with a road map for where we want to go. Then, like an archer with his arrow trained on the target, we can take aim. The effort is half completed once you've made the decision where to aim. Whether you decide to travel to the next town, or a faraway city, once you know where you are going, you just pack your bags, get in the car, and head in that direction. It's quite different from wandering aimlessly, unsure of where you are headed.

I cannot do anything unless I can dream and imagine it first. Can I imagine myself in a particular situation? Then I can probably do it. When my daughter was trying to figure out what to do with her life, which is not easy to know when you are in your twenties, I told her, "If it's something you enjoy and can see yourself doing five years down the line, it's probably the right thing." She thought I was crazy; to be able to imagine five years down the line seemed impossible. Five years was a lifetime for her. But when you are older, you know five years is a very short time. When I have a goal, I usually aim toward five years. It is my particular magic number; if I can imagine myself still interested or challenged five years down the road, then it helps me to choose what I'm going to do.

When we are younger, we are often naïve and without direction, throwing ourselves at life without any concept of what it will take to get there. Now we have more raw material to work with and can see more possibilities. As a mature person, we have a sense of the workload required, so the decisions are stronger and clearer. They're not taken lightly, but at the same time, they can be more fun.

If you don't know how to connect with your dreams, start by making a list. Write down what you think you are capable of doing. Listen to your inner voice: Ask yourself what excites you, what are you passionate about, then narrow it down to what actually makes sense. (I would probably rule out the roles of rocket scientist and astronaut, for instance.)

My sister Dari has talked about being a lawyer since she was a young girl. She had children early, so her dream was put on hold, but she kept it tucked away on the back shelf. Meanwhile she raised three kids, started a company, and helped all sorts of women's groups (my sister is the original feminist). One day she finally took that dream down from the shelf and dusted it off and is now enrolled in her second semester of law school. It took courage to hold on so long, but now she is fulfilling her dream.

Even (especially) at midlife, it's vital to have an inner vision. And it's never too late to act upon it. It is easy to tap into your passion simply through dreaming. So go for walks and contemplate, write those lists and meditate. Dreaming is your time to be creative about your potential and to move away from negativity. Dreaming helps you access what and where you want to be. Your dream is a flight to possibility and excitement. So dare to dream, have the courage to dream. And wait for the magic to happen.

Then whatever age you are you will have attained . . . Ageless Beauty.

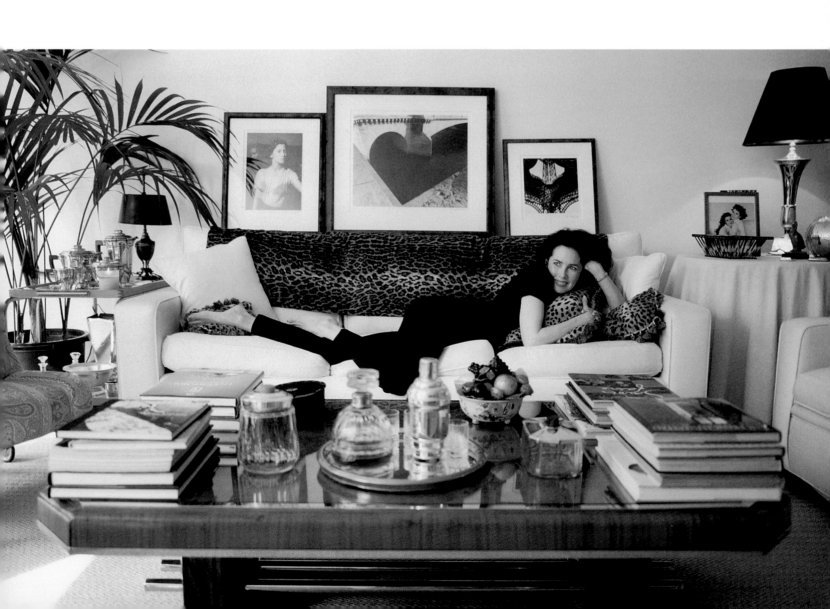

I LOVE THE AGE
I'M BECOMING

More than ever, I feel my life is an ongoing adventure. I feel more interest in what happens today than what was yesterday. And I am excited about the future and the possibilities it will bring; possibilities fueled by the experiences that have made up my life. Experiences I can draw on as I move forward.

In one generation, a world of possibilities has opened up to women. Now, as the enormous number of baby boomers start to hit fifty, we are demanding a different quality of life and have the sheer numbers to make a difference. Our eyes are open to the choices that lie ahead and instead of feeling resignation, we are open to our potential for another thirty, forty, even fifty terrific years of living life to the fullest, enjoying good looks—and good health.

I have told you what is important to me, shared my story—shared my secrets. And now I would love to hear from you. My dream—and my goal—is to exchange information and wisdom with women around the world and discover what you have learned over the years. I would love to hear about your hopes, achievements, philosophy, insights—and what you have to tell me about health, beauty, and well-being. (Because I'm still learning, learning, learning, too.)

Let us create a forum where our experiences can be pooled and shared, because we all have so much to give to each other. So please, accept this invitation. Write to me by letter or e-mail at www.dayle.com. Share what's touched you in your life and what you have learned along the way. And please join me in the celebration.

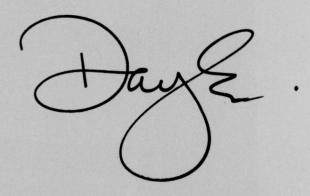

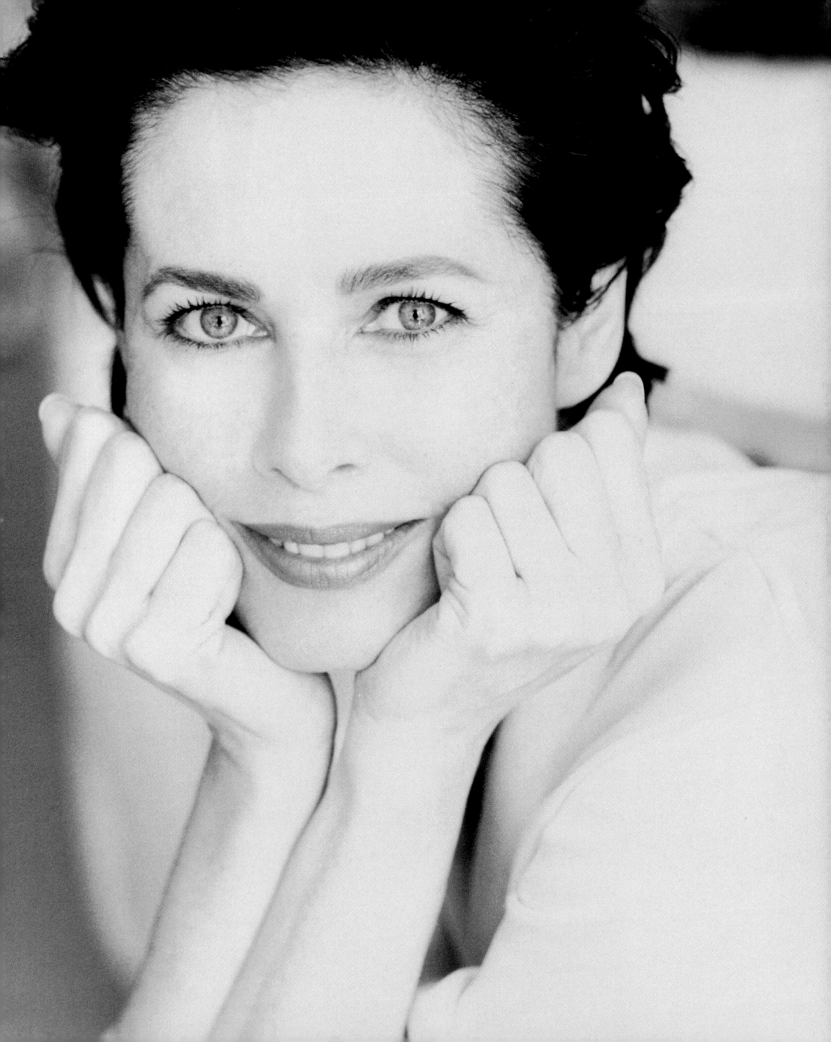

RESOURCES

CHAPTER 1: FACE REALITY

1.	Eric Javits Hats	(800) 374-HATS
2.	Frownies–Vermont Country Store	(800) 362-0405
3.	Flaxseed Eye Pillow–Vermont Country Store	(800) 362-0405
4.	Cell Tech	(800) 800-1300
5.	Tongue Cleaner	(888) 264-YOGA
6.	American Academy of Cosmetic Dentistry (AACD)	(800) 543-9220
7.	The American Society for Dental Aesthetics	(800) 454-ASDA
8.	International Guild of Professional Electrologists	(800) 830-3247

CHAPTER 2: FABULOUS FACE MAKING MAKEUP

1.	Japanese rice powder–Shu Uemura	(888) 540-8181
2.	Face Stockholm	(800) 334-FACE
3.	Francois Nars	(888) 903-NARS
4.	Tweezerman Tweezers	(800) 645-3340
5.	Ilise Harris eyelash curler	(914) 674-6645
6.	Make Up For Ever gloss	(800) 757-5175
7.	Zitomer's Pharmacy	(212) 737-4480

CHAPTER 3: CONFIDENCE-BOOSTING HAIR

1.	Philip B. Hair & Skin Care	(800) 643-5556
2.	Stephen Knoll Hair Products	(800) 728-7822
3.	Phyto Hair Care Products	(800) 55PHYTO
4.	Kiehl's Hair & Skin Care	(800) 543-4571
5.	Frederic Fekkai Hair Products	(888) FFEKKAI

CHAPTER 4: BODY TALK

1.	Agave cloths–Zitomer's Pharmacy	(212) 737-4480

CHAPTER 5: EXERCISE: DON'T SWEAT IT!

1.	Sony "Voice File"	(888) 987-7669
2.	Trapeze Arts	(415) 3317-1900 or www.trapezeart.com
3.	Pilates	(800) 474-5283 or (888) 474-5283
4.	Lotte Berk Method (studios in NY & CT)	NY(212) 288-6613 CT(203)661-4163
5.	Mini trampoline (Legacy International, Inc.)	(800) 651-3622

CHAPTER 6: THINK THINNER: MIDDLE-AGE SPREAD IS NOT A GIVEN

1.	Eco Pump–California Olive Oil Corporation	(508) 745-7840; Fax (508) 744-3492
2.	Wax Orchard "Oh Fudge"	22744 Wax Orchards Rd, SW, Vashon, WA 98070
3.	Balance Bars	(800) 678-4246
4.	WAKE CUP–Whole Earth Foods, Ltd. Belgravia Imports, Newport, RI	(401) 849-1122
7.	CALI TEA by Sunrider	(212) 872-2650

CHAPTER 7: STRESS BUSTING

1.	Bionaire humidifier	(800) 253-2764

Spas:

2.	Bliss Spa	(212) 219-8970
3.	The Peninsula Spa	(212) 903-3910
4.	Susan Ciminelli Day Spa	(212) 872-2650
5.	Canyon Ranch	(800) 742-9000
6.	The Golden Door	(800) 424-0777

CHAPTER 8: HEALTHY MIND, HEALTHY YOU

1.   One to One/The National Mentoring Partnership is an organization that can put you in touch with any of over 100 mentoring programs. 2801 M Street NW, Washington DC, 20007. telephone (202) 338-3844; fax (202) 338-1642

2.   Green Chimneys is an organization that helps children at risk by giving them the responsibility of caring for abused animals. (914) 279-2995 ext. 102

3.   Big Brothers Big Sisters of America (215) 567-7000 will put you in touch with local branch

4.	Youth Mentoring Program Directory	United Way of America catalog # UN10662 (800) 772-0008
5.	Agraria potpourri	(415) 863-7700
6.	Santa Maria Novella potpourri Takashimaya Department Store in NY	(800) 753-2038

CHAPTER 9: LIVING AND LONGEVITY

1.	National Mental Information Health Center	(800) 969-NMHA

2.   Michelle Bernhardt is a renowned metaphysical consultant who brings new awareness and new meaning to people's lives. (800) 760-5452

3.	Spa Finders	Spa Finders.com (800) All-SPAS

CATALOG NUMBERS

Garnet Hill	(800) 622-6216
The Company Store	(800) 285-3696
Chambers	(800) 334-9790
Lands End	(800) 356-4444
Hold Everything	(800) 421-2264
Coming Home	(800) 345-3696
The Sharper Image	(800) 344-5555
The Vermont Country Store	(802) 362-0405

SUGGESTED READING LIST

Ageless Body, Timeless Mind. Deepak Chopra (Harmony Books)

The Beauty Myth. Naomi Wolfe (Anchor)

The Complete Book of Juicing. Michael T. Murray (Prima Publishing)

Creative Caring. Beth Kitzinger, Linda Davies Rocky (Wildcat Canyon Press)

Fire with Fire. Naomi Wolfe (Fawcett Columbine)

Gift from the Sea. Anne Morrow Lindbergh (Pantheon Books)

Handbook for the Soul. Richard Carlson, Benjamin Shields (Little, Brown)

Healing Foods. Miriam Polunin (Dorling Kindersley)

How to Heal Depression. Harold Bloomfield, Peter McWilliams (Prelude Press)

How to Survive the Loss of a Love. Melba Colgrove, Harold Bloomfield, Peter
    McWilliams (Prelude Press)

Natural Healing for Women. Susan Curtis & Ronny Fraser (Thorsons Books)

Natural Medicine for Women. Julian & Susan Scott (Avon Books)

Natural Woman, Natural Menopause. Marcus Laux, Christine Conrad
    (HarperCollins)

Openings. Shelly Tucker (Whiteaker Press)

Passages. Gail Sheehy (Random House)

The Power of Beauty. Nancy Friday (HarperCollins)

Promiscuities. Naomi Wolf (Random House)

The Rest of Us. Jacquelyn Mitchard (Viking Press)

Revolution from Within. Gloria Steinem (Little, Brown)

The Second Sex. Simone de Beauvoir

She. Robert Johnson (HarperSanFrancisco)

The Silent Passage: Menopause. Gail Sheehy (Random House)

Simple Abundance. Sarah Ban Breathnach (Warner Books)

T'ai Ji for Beginners. Chungliag Al Huang (Celestial Arts Publications)

Ten Principles of Spiritual Parenting. Mimi Doe (HarperPerennial)

The Ways of the Mystic. Joan Borysenko (Hay House)

Welcome to Your Facelift. Helen Bransford (Doubleday)

A Woman's Book of Life. Joan Borysenko (Riverhead Books)

A Woman's Guide to a Better Life. Andrea Van Steinhouse (Three Rivers Press)

PHOTO CREDITS

cover
  Patrick Demarchelier

2 left to right
  Ilan Rubin
  Francine Fleischer
  Ilan Rubin
  Carlton Davis
  Javier Vallhonrat
  Ilan Rubin
  Maria Robledo
  Michel Comte

3 left to right
  Gentl & Hyers
    courtesy of
    W Magazine
  Gentl & Hyers/
    Photonica
  Torkil Gudnason
  Maria Robledo
  Enrique Badulescu
  Toni Thorimbert
  Gentl & Hyers
  Arthur Elgort

6 Guy Bourdin

8 Francine Fleischer

11 left to right from top
  Michel Comte
  Arthur Elgort
  Michael McDermott
  Mark Bugzester
  Michelle McCabe
  Michel Comte
  Arthur Elgort
  Michel Comte
  Michel Comte
  Victor Skrebneski
  Andre Rau
  Francine Fleischer
  Michel Comte
  Michel Comte
  J.J.
  Troy Word

12 Peggy Sirota

15 clockwise
  Oberto Gili
  Andre Rau
  Andre Rau
  Francine Fleischer
  Andre Rau
  Lumi
  Troy Word

16 Jonathan Kantor

18 Amy Van Dyken
  photographed for
  Tag Heuer's launch
  of its new sports
  watch Kirium

21 Torkil Gudnason

22 Troy Word

23 Cindy Palmano

24 Andre Rau

26 Yasutaka Tanji

27 Raymond Meier

29 Jonathan Kantor

32 Patrick Demarchelier
    courtesy of
    Harper's Bazaar

33 Troy Word

34 left to right
  Richard Bocklet/Sipa
  Rickerby/Sipa
  Scott Brinegar/Sipa
  Fred Prouser/Sipa

35 Oberto Gili

36 Carlton Davis

37 top to bottom
  Photofest
  Fred Prouser/Sipa
  Aslan, Sutcliffe/Sipa
  Aslan, Sutcliffe/Sipa
  Culver Pictures
  David Niviere/Sipa
  Photofest
  Niviere, Barthelemy,
    Villard/Sipa
  Antoine Verglas
  Photofest

38 Enrique Badulescu

41 Toni Thorimbert

43 Mario Testino

44 Ilan Rubin

49 Javier Vallhonrat

50 Troy Word

52 Troy Word

53 Troy Word

54 Troy Word

55 Francine Fleischer

57 Troy Word

58 Troy Word

59 Franicine Fleischer

60 Torkil Gudnason

63 Carlton Davis

64 clockwise
    from top left
  Ilan Rubin
  Ilan Rubin
  Ilan Rubin
  Raymond Meier

65 Ilan Rubin

66 Michelle McCabe

67 Andre Rau

68 Andre Rau

69 Michael McDermott
  (both)

71 Ilan Rubin

72 Troy Word

73 top to bottom
  Photofest
  Alberto Tolot/Outline
  Culver Pictures
  Arthur Elgort
  Russel Wong/Outline
  Stephen Danelian/
    Outline
  Georges Rech
  Sutcliffe/Sipa
  Deborah Feingold/
    Outline
  Michael Daks/Outline

74 Maria Robledo (both)

77 Ilan Rubin (all)

79 Francine Fleischer

82 Ilan Rubin

85 Michelle McCabe

87 Patrick Demarchelier

88 Troy Word

89 Jonathan Kantor

90 Ilan Rubin

91 Ilan Rubin

92 Antoine Verglas

96 Gentl & Hyers

97 Javier Vallhonrat

98 Jonathan Kantor

100 Troy Word (all)

102 top to bottom
  Culver Pictures
  Culver Pictures
  Culver Pictures
  Photofest

106 Jonathan Kantor (all)

109 Enrique Badulescu

110 Troy Word

111 Miles Aldridge

114 Stephen Anderson

117 Troy Word (all)

118 Enrique Badulescu

122 Arthur Elgort (all)

125 Javier Vallhonrat

126 Michelle McCabe

130 Ilan Rubin

132 TBD

136 Jonathan Kantor

141 Carlton Davis

142 Jonathan Kantor

144 MacDuff Everton

147 Ilan Rubin

148 Antoine Verglas

149 Torkil Gudnason

152 Toni Thorimbert

153 Jonathan Kantor

155 Gentl & Hyers
    courtesy of
    W Magazine

157 Javier Vallhonrat

159 Javier Vallhonrat

160 Gilles Bensimon

162 Maria Robledo

165 Javier Vallhonrat

166 Michel Comte

167 Michel Comte

168 Victor Skrebneski

169 Chris Nicholls

170 Michel Comte

172 top to bottom
  Torkil Gudnason
  Torkil Gudnason
  Jonathan Kantor
  Jonathan Kantor

174 Maria Robledo

175 Jonathan Kantor

177 Carlton Davis

179 Maria Robledo (both)

181 Javier Vallhonrat

183 Gentl & Hyers
    courtesy of
    W Magazine

184 Troy Word

185 Gentl & Hyers/
    Photonica

186 Maria Robledo

188 Torkil Gudnason

190 Enrique Badulescu

191 Javier Vallhonrat

194 Gentl & Hyers/
    Photonica

196 Ilan Rubin

200 Javier Vallhonrat

201 Oberto Gili

203 YanN Gamblin

205 Andre Rau

back cover - left to right
    from upper left
  Oberto Gili
  Torkil Gudnason
  MacDuff Everton
  Andre Rau
  Gentl & Hyers/
    Photonica
  Torkil Gudnason
  Carlton Davis
  Maria Robledo
  Javier Vallhonrat
  Javier Vallhonrat
  Enrique Badulescu

Thanks to:
Sandy Linter
Bryan Marryshow
Patti Trujillo
Marty Hamilton
Jorge Serio
Ringo
Vesna Brozovic
Kimbra Kierulff
Rick Pipino
John Rosen @ Nucleus
  (printing/retouching)

A special thanks for their
  generosity with photo
  archives:
Town & Country
Harper's Bazaar
Maska